THE END OF AGEING

THE END OF AGEING

HOW BIOTECHNOLOGY IS
REDEFINING HUMAN LIFE AND
WHAT IT MEANS FOR US

THOMAS RAMGE

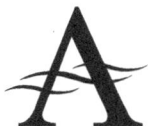

ANTHEM PRESS

Anthem Press
An imprint of Wimbledon Publishing Company
www.anthempress.com

This edition first published in UK and USA 2025
by ANTHEM PRESS
75–76 Blackfriars Road, London SE1 8HA, UK
or PO Box 9779, London SW19 7ZG, UK
and
244 Madison Ave #116, New York, NY 10016, USA

British Library Cataloguing-in-Publication Data
A catalogue record for this book is available from the British Library.

Library of Congress Cataloging-in-Publication Data: 2025932547
A catalog record for this book has been requested.

ISBN-13: 978-1-83999-555-2 (Pbk)
ISBN-10: 1-83999-555-6 (Pbk)

Cover Credit: Designed by dgim-studio / Freepik

This title is also available as an e-book.

CONTENTS

It is one of the most remarkable things that in all of the biological sciences there is no clue as to the necessity of death. If you say we want to make perpetual motion, we have discovered enough laws as we studied physics to see that it is either absolutely impossible or else the laws are wrong.

But there is nothing in biology yet found that indicates the inevitability of death. This suggests to me that it is not at all inevitable, and that it is only a matter of time before the biologists discover what it is that is causing us the trouble and that that terrible universal disease or temporariness of the human's body will be cured.

Richard Feynman, Nobel laureate and physicist, 1964

Death is the destination we all share. No one has ever escaped it. And that is as it should be. Because death is very likely the single best invention of life. It's life's change agent, it clears out the old to make way for the new.

Right now the new is you. But someday not too long from now, you will gradually become the old and be cleared away. Sorry to be so dramatic. But it's quite true.

Your time is limited. So don't waste it living someone else's life. Don't be trapped by dogma, which is living with the results of other people's thinking. Don't let the noise of others opinions drown out your own inner voice.

Steve Jobs, Stanford Commencement Speech, 2005

ABOUT THE AUTHOR

Dr. Thomas Ramge has authored more than 20 books on science, technology, and innovation and how they change the way we live, work, and think.

His essays and long-read articles are published in *MIT Management Review, Harvard Business Review, Foreign Affairs, The Economist, Die Zeit, Frankfurter Allgemeine Zeitung, Die Welt*, among others. He has received numerous book and journalism awards, including the Axiom Business Book Award (Gold Medal Economics), the Best Business Book Award on Innovation and Technology, the getAbstract International Book Award, the German Business Book Award, the German Essay Prize, and the Herbert Quandt Media Award.

Thomas is an associated researcher at the Einstein Center Digital Future and host of the podcast SPRIND by the Federal Agency for Breakthrough Innovation of Germany. He lives in Berlin with his wife and son.

ACKNOWLEDGEMENTS

The decision to write this book came after a lecture on longevity at the Weberbank Berlin in the spring of 2022. The audience's reactions were so emotional; the discussions that followed were so lively and yet profound that I decided to dive much deeper into the topic of biotechnical life extension. I thank the Weberbank and Christian Bracht for organizing the evening of 'Eternal Life'. And I thank my friend and colleague Christoph Koch, who gave me the first impulse to deal with the topic through a joint podcast.

For invaluable scientific insights, I thank the many, many researchers and experts who granted me their time in recent years for interviews and background conversations. Too many names to name, and if I started, I would run the risk of forgetting too many. As an exception, I do want to mention Dr Karl Schlagenhauf, a senior biotech expert of the Federal Agency for Breakthrough Innovation, who patiently explained the complex processes in cells and checked the technical chapter for errors.

But above all, I would like to thank you, dear readers, for your interest in this book and for the time you spend on it. We are still mortal. And time is still precious. 🙏

PREQUEL: A DAY IN THE LIFE OF A 200-YEAR-OLD

This summer I will be 200 years old. I'm really looking forward to the birthday party. I'm sure there will be more than five hundred guests, including many of my great-great-great-grandchildren. Of course, they can't imagine what life was like in 2025 when I was born. My statistical life expectancy back then was around eighty years. At least that's how the statistics department of the National Health Service calculated it back then based on the mortality tables of the time. Of course, anyone who was intensively involved in molecular biology and biomedicine in the mid-20s of the twenty-first century did not believe in such a pessimistic prognosis. My parents were very interested in all approaches to longevity medicine and tried to optimize their lifestyle for the longest possible lifespan: low-calorie diet, exercise, healthy sleep, the usual. My mum also took medication, which was considered a sensible addition to a healthy lifestyle in the longevity scene at the time. Also the usual: statins to keep the cardiovascular system going, rapamycin in the hope of improving cell renewal and reducing inflammation.

Unfortunately, my parents won't be able to come to my birthday. My father died in 2039, when I was a teenager, in a car accident caused by an idiot who thought he had to switch off the autopilot, which was against the law. Perhaps the early death of my father contributed to the fact that, as a student, I agreed to take part in the first major clinical trials for life extension. My mum was also allowed to take part. She lived to the age of 110 and was largely healthy until 107. But the therapies started too late for her to achieve true agelessness. I was lucky in timing. And I belong to the first generation of the truly long-lived, because my body was still young when I was given the first really potent longevity drugs. Since then, I haven't aged biologically. But what exactly does luck mean here? Luck does not equal happiness.

As predicted, when biomedical breakthroughs are achieved, an extremely long life is of course an ambivalent endeavour. The Flying Dutchman already knew that. At least one thing we know for sure today: when biotechnology redefines life, everything changes.

Let's start with social relationships. Today, there are around ten thousand double-centenarians, as scientists call us, worldwide. There are only a very few of us who have spent the majority of our lives with one spouse. Most of us have found a life model in which we spend one to three decades with a partner and then move on to new shores. I myself have had nine serious relationships so far. I reached my ethically agreed limit of three children at 110. Here in the UK, limiting the number of children for long-lifers is rather a commitment, not a legal obligation. I abide by it because the danger of planetary overpopulation naturally increases with every new cohort of long-lifers. Hence, I haven't felt any desire to have children for decades, because I have over fifty descendants and a good relationship with most of them.

I find it very enriching that I am no longer perceived as old, but as experienced. You can even see that on the football pitch. I can still keep up physically, but of course I can read the game better than the mentally young ones. Overall, I find family relationships more relaxed than my parents always described them to me. I feel less obligated. Bonds are more flexible and pragmatic, and that must be the case because we have so many more social relationships these days. Family has become more dynamic, more open to new constellations and, therefore, in my perception, more honest. I find that a huge gain in the quality of life.

In turn, I am burdened by the fact that I have, of course, seen many old companions die who have decided against longevity medicine. Fortunately, all my children are long-lifers, and none of them have had an accident or a still-incurable illness. The funerals of some of my grandchildren and great-grandchildren, on the other hand, have been the biggest psychological burden of my life so far. Sometimes I ask myself: How many blows of fate can an old soul withstand?

I am still mentally healthy, and I do a lot to keep it that way, including intensive discussions with my AI psychologist, who has been with me for more than fifty years. But still, sometimes it feels like time doesn't heal all wounds. Some of my long-lived friends have chosen suicide in the middle of their second century. I don't think they have managed to improve their ability to grieve and say goodbye. Even if it may sound a little brutal, in order to safeguard our mental health, we long-lifers must learn to draw clearer lines than normal mortals. There are simply many more chapters that we have to close in order to be able to open new ones. That's why we sometimes seem unsympathetic, even selfish, to ordinary mortals. I can understand it, but I believe that the ability to separate does not necessarily have to lead to overly self-centred character traits or even maliciousness. This is how long-lived characters were generally portrayed in literature before long-lived people actually existed. Hence, psychological studies on us long-lived people tend to point to an interesting ambivalence. On the one hand, an above-average number of people who opted for longevity therapies consider themselves to be 'above average important'.

The technical term for this is narcissist self-selection. But this is clearly only one side of the coin.

In my perception, many long-lifers develop a milder view of their own lives, their fellow human beings, and therefore also social issues after the first biologically regular life cycle at the latest. Yes, there are quite a few first-person shooter types among us. They don't seem particularly happy to me. On the other hand, there are many who take more time to get deeply involved and connected with others. We have enough time. There is also a technical term for this: longevity mellowness. Of course, selfishness and altruism are not mutually exclusive anyway and certainly not in a very long life. To be honest, I myself only started volunteering intensively when I could no longer cope with the boredom in my life.

Deadly boredom in a life without death was, self-evidently, predicted by many authors of the nineteenth and twentieth centuries. Not knowing what to do with ample time was the enemy we saw coming. The interim assessment of us long-lifers here is mixed. The finite nature of life has made and continues to make ordinary mortals realize that time is precious. We often find it difficult to really savour the moments. There are at least two psychological mechanisms behind this that are difficult to switch off. Without time pressure, we are less likely to consciously create moments of concentrated happiness, or even unconsciously work towards them. Not putting things off is a real problem and the inner bastard has become an even tougher opponent. And when we do experience these moments of concentrated happiness in a later phase of life, they don't feel like 'the first time'. Happiness then comes round the corner as an old acquaintance. Nice that you're here, but no reason to be euphoric. Some long-lived people therefore consciously try to erase old experiences from their memory, some even with medication. They then experience new things more often, but at the cost of consciously robbing themselves of their own identity. I ask myself: Are these people actually still the same person they were born as? I belong to the group that deliberately tries to reinvent itself again and again without cutting its own roots. On the contrary, I consciously try to use my long-life experience to reach new levels of excellence in new domains. At least in my professional career, I have managed to do this quite well.

My first degree in the 2040s was in mechanical engineering. I may have followed my parents' advice and wishes. Looking back, it wasn't a bad decision. I was able to make a small contribution to the electromagnetic heat chambers for nuclear fusion finally becoming a reality. Nuclear fusion has been providing clean, too-cheap-to-metre energy for everyone since 2070. I was proud of the achievement, but then it really was time for a fresh professional start. As a 20-year-old, I didn't dare to study maths, but at 55 I did. I didn't become a top mathematician in my second career either, but it was enough to become an AI systems manager for a large insurance company. After 15 years, however, that actually became too boring for me. I then felt real fulfilment, at least for three decades, as a live musician. The magic of live music hasn't really changed, nor has the fact that the wages for most musicians have remained meagre. I was certainly privileged in this respect: when I was touring the clubs, I simply lived off the returns on my savings that I was able to build up as an engineer and actuary. Unfortunately, this came to an end around the turn of the twenty-second century.

With each new generation of long-lifers, the central banks had to lower key interest rates, otherwise public finances would have gone completely off the rails. Pension payments were suspended for us long-lifers anyway, when the first of us could actually have retired. Most of us will have to work for as long as our health allows. So perhaps forever.

I was a carpenter for a short time in my second century, a teacher for a long time, and now a doctor for young mortals for more than twenty-five years. If we can cure a seriously ill mortal person, I usually try to convince them to undergo longevity therapy. Even today, this only works if the body has not yet shown any major signs of wear and tear. Sometimes the choice for longevity treatment still fails because of financial means, although the therapies have become significantly cheaper in recent decades and are also more accessible in middle-income countries. The right to longevity treatment only exists in a few rich countries, such as Saudi Arabia, Singapore, Switzerland, and Bangladesh. On the other hand, economists have coined a neat term for the societal benefits of life extension: the longevity dividend. The monthly cost of health insurance for long-lifers has fallen drastically. Our biologically young bodies are simply much less often ill, at least physically.

As a doctor, I learn something new every day, both professionally and personally. For me, that is the best medicine against the fast-time effect many long-lifers suffer from. For them, time flies faster every year. So, what is an additional year worth for them? I feel this coming, too. It might be time for a new challenge soon. But not all long-lifers are looking for regular change.

I know scientists who can now look back on 150 years of experience in their discipline. And the best of them manage not to remain trapped in their mental ruts but instead use their expertise to recognize where the opportunity for something new is lurking. These super experts are perhaps the greatest resource of our time. Without them, I was sceptical that we will be able to master the great challenges of our time: growing inequality and a rapidly growing world population. Perhaps the greatest danger today, however, is to bring those long-lifers to their senses who are not aware of the individual responsibility that longevity entails for societies and humanity.

CHAPTER 1

DO YOU WANT TO LIVE FOREVER?

Let's do a thought experiment. Tomorrow, your physician offers you a choice of three pills: a white, a yellow, or a green one.

The white pill allows you to live in good health to 100. With luck and good genes, you will even live to 110. No cancer, no pain, no Alzheimer's. In the end, you will die the way most of us want to pass away today – without prolonged suffering, fear, or knowing exactly when death will come.

If you choose the yellow pill, you will live in the best health to be around 200 years – at least as old as a giant tortoise. If things go particularly well, you could also reach the age of a Greenland shark, so between 400 and 500 years.

Through the centuries, your body will hardly age. You will always feel good and have the physical and mental capacity as today during the second quarter of life between the ages of 20 and 40. Once the first signs of ageing emerge, you will get another yellow pill. But like the giant tortoise or the Greenland shark, you will eventually die. This death would also be peaceful.

The green medication gives you eternal physical life. Although you cannot rule out with certainty that you will eventually die in an industrial accident, this is becoming increasingly unlikely due to technical progress and better safety features in all domains of life. You will live in a world where medical progress is faster than natural ageing. In this scenario, the new medication is also more powerful than new diseases that arise in the Earth's biosphere. We will have 'longevity escape velocity', as the bioinformatician Aubrey de Grey calls it. The (individual) human being's life expectancy increases by more than one year yearly. Death is defeated. We can live forever, but we don't have to.

As in the second scenario, you can also choose suicide as an exit option for the green pill so you won't be trapped in an immortal body. Therefore, you do not have to be bored to death in infinite loops of repetition like Raymond Fosca, the immortal and unhappy hero in Simone de Beauvoir's novel *Tous les hommes sont mortels* (*All Men Are Mortal*) from 1946. I call this scenario 'Highlander with suicide option'. The older ones (by today's standards) may remember the title song of the film *Highlander* by the group Queen: 'Who Wants to Live Forever?'

The singer Freddie Mercury died shortly after that of HIV, which evolution had only just produced.

Which option would you choose?

1. White pill: 'Like today, only better'
2. Yellow pill: 'The Greenland shark scenario'
3. Green pill: 'Highlander with suicide option'

I often play this thought experiment with participants in my lectures and workshops. They are supposed to choose as quickly as possible, and their intuition should be the (co-)decider.

Almost always, the majority votes for the familiar and easy to imagine: Please, give me the white pill! Play it safe. Experiencing health at 95 and seeing how your grandchildren find their path in life, perhaps holding a great-grandchild in your arms and then falling asleep gently – that would be it.

In most of these groups, more people choose the Greenland shark option than eternity. The reasoning for this could be: life is too short. You would like to be able to think outside the constraints of time, but at some point, it's enough. Many participants also say that the turtle's time is actually enough. It does not have to be 400 years.

Choosing the Greenland shark scenario doesn't really make sense in purely rational decision-making. The immortal with an option for suicide can downgrade his life to scenario 2 at any time. But even in this thought experiment, a decision about life possibilities and death is, of course, not a purely rational decision. The idea of killing oneself arouses unsettling feelings in many people, even if suicide may still be many centuries into the future. Who knows if you will even find the courage to end your life, even if suffering is too much? It is less difficult to leave the final decision to fate or biology.

Who chooses scenario 3? Usually, it's participants who characterize themselves as particularly optimistic. Often, they are science fiction fans. They like books, films, and computer games in which, thanks to science and technology, the old myths of the fountain of youth and the philosopher's stone will become a reality in the future – at least in fiction. Many of these technology optimists know that immortality, with or without an exit option, is, despite all the advances in biotechnology, still science fiction, at least today.

No one can rule out one hundred per cent that someone will actually invent a green pill in the indeterminate future. It is radical innovation's nature that such advances are literally unpredictable. After all, as thinking and researching beings, we don't know what we can't know, but what a genius of our species – or more likely a team of scientific geniuses – might eventually find out. The green pill is theoretically possible. However, as things stand today, no discernible scientific and technological development path makes immortality even remotely likely. This no longer applies to scenarios 1 and 2. It is plausible that they will become a reality in our lifetime.

Medicine in Attack Mode

Molecular biologists and biomedical scientists, geneticists, and gerontologists, supported by computer scientists and AI scientists, understand the blueprint of life better and better. They increase their knowledge of why and how cells, organs, and organisms age as a whole system and how you can significantly slow down this ageing process. Sometimes you can stop and even reverse this ageing process in certain experiments and for specific cell types. Life sciences as a whole will increase the realistic chance of pushing back death as we know it in the coming decades. With a bit of luck, skill, and many billions of dollars spent in research, it can be possible to radically weaken and, in some cases, even defeat age-related diseases – the malignant harbingers of death. Plausible scenarios also include breaking the glass ceiling of the human age of around 120 years, and people could continue to live healthy lives for a few more decades.

Possible active ingredients of white and yellow pills from our thought experiment are already effective in animals. They are sometimes even clinically tested on humans. Approved gene therapies are rapidly increasing the knowledge base for longevity medicine. Of course, this does not mean that significant breakthroughs are imminent. Medical advances against ageing will likely take longer than the founders and venture capitalists of the corresponding biotech start-ups claim. Something similar was often observed in the past when new technologies made their challenging way into the world, and their developers and financiers turned up their marketing efforts as much as possible. Occasionally, however, scientific and technological innovations also lead to significant changes in the present faster than many experts suspected. It was the same with artificial fertilizers, penicillin, or the mainframe computer.

'The only way of discovering the limits of the possible is to venture a little way past them to the impossible', writes science fiction author Arthur M. Clarke. In the life sciences, scientific boundaries – that no one knew existed 40 or 50 years ago – have been transcended in the last two decades. It is time for us individuals and societies to deal in-depth with the biomedical progress of what scientists call 'longevity', because medicine is currently switching from defensive to attack mode against death. What does this mean?

In the last 150 years, the average life expectancy globally has more than doubled. In the United States, the life expectancy of a child born in the late nineteenth century was about 40. That's hardly more than in the Stone Age or the Middle Ages. US-Americans today have a statistical life expectancy of about 80 years, French and Italians 82, and Japanese more than 84 years. Societies with lower per capita income have caught up significantly in statistical life expectancy in recent decades. The average life expectancy worldwide today is around 73 years. Every year since 1950, the average life expectancy around the world has risen by 18 weeks.

The enormous increase in average life expectancy was achieved above all because science, technology, and culture systematically combated the causes of early death, particularly infant mortality and infectious diseases. In 1800, almost half of all newborns in the United States did not make it to their fifth birthday. In 2022, it was only about seven out of a thousand. In Canada, Australia, Japan, South Korea, and European countries, child mortality is even significantly lower. At the beginning of the twentieth century, about half of all US citizens died of pneumonia, tuberculosis, or diarrhoea. It is only 3 per cent today, thanks to antibiotics, antivirals, and hygiene practices. In the second half of the twentieth century and the last two and a half decades, medicine developed better therapies for diseases such as cardiovascular disease (CVD), type 2 diabetes, and many cancers, which often shorten life in the second half of life. Healthier lifestyles, better nutrition, and more exercise contribute to extending our life span, of course not for everyone but statistically.

From a conventional medical point of view, the most important characteristic of ageing is that the probability of getting sick and dying from a disease increases exponentially throughout our lives. The defensive mode systematically eliminates illnesses as causes of death. This allows us to raise average life expectancy. But the catch is: we are not getting to grips with death at an advanced age. While the number of centenarians is slowly growing, only 1 in 1,000 of them celebrates their 110th birthday. And no one in history has made it beyond 125. With

Inah Canabarro Lucas aged 116 (in March 2025) being the oldest person alive, this won't change any time soon. Meanwhile, it is crystal clear that to break the biological glass ceiling of 120 or so years, medical research needs to switch to attack mode.

The development of life expectancy is as gratifying as it is impressive. But it also has a downside: evolution has not genetically optimized humans (like most other mammals) to live healthily for 80 to 100 years. The gene mutation selection mechanism determines with statistical precision that a virus would have killed our ancestors by the age of 50 or 60 at the latest. They would have been eaten by the sabre-toothed tiger or killed by another human being. In the biology of evolution, it made sense to equip the genus *Homo sapiens* with a body capable of bringing up their children by the age of 30 to 40.

It is helpful for the genus when grandmothers are still around to help raise the grandchildren. For this reason, women are likely to have a higher life expectancy than men. But why should evolution in humans select mutations in which teeth grow back many times, as in the Greenland shark? A set of teeth that lasts into the fifth decade should be enough. Why should a cell be able to divide or renew hundreds or even thousands of times when a few dozen cell divisions are enough for a lifetime?

The giant tortoise from scenario 2 offers a striking counterexample. Their shell protects them so well from enemies that in the millions of years of their evolution, genes have prevailed that make their organism long-living and reproductive for a much longer life span. A 150-year-old turtle carries about the same risk of dying in the coming year as a 25-year-old turtle. Biologically speaking, the 1,000-pound colossus is ageless. For us humans, on the other hand, the risk of death increases drastically with increasing age. An 80-year-old person has a 60 times higher risk of death than a 30-year-old. Medically, age is the highest risk factor. A chain-smoking, overweight 40-year-old alcoholic might have, in most circumstances, a much better chance of celebrating his next birthday than an athletic abstainer at 80.

From the viewpoint of an elderly, frail person with a strict will to live healthily, that is quite deplorable. For evolution, this makes sense, as science writer Geoffrey Carr points out in an in-depth report on longevity medicine in *The Economist.* Evolution favours reproduction, not longevity. Why is that?

Life is shaped by both genes and the environment. But in the end, it's the environment – through accidents, predators, and diseases – that determines how long most creatures live. Genes that only provide benefits later in life, after an organism has likely already faced the dangers of its surroundings, aren't likely to thrive – unless they offer advantages in other ways. On the other hand, genes that contribute to a strong, healthy, and fertile youth are far more likely to succeed and spread.

In fact, evolution may even work against old age. If a gene helps an animal reproduce when it is young, but harms it later in life, natural selection is still likely to favour it. For example, some evidence suggests that a particular gene linked to Alzheimer's disease may provide reproductive advantages to younger individuals, even though it increases the risk of disease later in life.

From an evolutionary perspective, an individual organism exists primarily as a vehicle for passing on genes, rather than as an end in itself. Keeping the body in prime condition is only worthwhile if it increases the chances of passing on more genes to the next generation. If the resources required for repair and maintenance are better spent elsewhere – such as boosting early survival and reproduction – then the body's repair systems will naturally decline. This idea, known as the 'disposable soma' theory, suggests that once an organism is no longer useful for reproduction, it becomes expendable.

This explains why so many age-related diseases – such as Alzheimer's, Parkinson's, retinal degeneration, type 2 diabetes, and various cancers – are rare in youth but common in old age. However, this does not mean ageing is inevitable or irreversible. Evolution may not have prioritized long-term repair, but that doesn't mean we can't find ways to keep our bodies in good working order. With the right scientific insights and innovations, we may yet outsmart nature's original plan.

About 150,000 people die every day worldwide. 100,000 of them die 'of old age', as we call this colloquially. Medically speaking, they die of age-related diseases, which in turn are usually the result of cellular degeneration and resulting functional disorders of the body and brain.

Age-related diseases arise due to the gradual breakdown of cellular function. This process is driven by genetic programming, metabolic decline, and cumulative damage from oxidative stress and inflammation. Over time, the body's repair mechanisms weaken, making cells vulnerable to mutations, protein misfolding, and energy inefficiencies. This degeneration manifests as neurodegenerative disorders like Alzheimer's, CVDs due to arterial plaque buildup, and metabolic disorders such as type 2 diabetes. The brain, in particular, suffers from diminished neuronal plasticity, leading to cognitive decline, memory loss, and reduced ability to regulate bodily functions effectively.

Another key factor in ageing is the gradual shortening of telomeres, the protective caps on the ends of chromosomes. With each cell division, telomeres shorten until cells can no longer divide, leading to tissue degradation and organ failure. This process, combined with chronic inflammation, contributes to muscle loss, immune system decline, and increased vulnerability to infections. The accumulation of non-functional, senescent cells further exacerbates these issues, releasing harmful inflammatory signals that accelerate age-related decline.

So far, these mechanisms have been viewed as medically inevitable. But are they indeed?

Is Death a Disease?

The great successes that the defensive mode can demonstrate have a downside. Because we have succeeded so well in the last century and a half in systematically eliminating the formerly relevant causes of death, we are now suffering more and more from those that have evolutionarily been designed as degeneration in the human body. We buy the longer life that hygiene and medical progress allow us with suffering in old age because medicine simply cannot stop degeneration – the increasing accumulation of damage in the cells in the later decades of life. To put it even more bluntly: We have only slightly slowed down ageing but significantly prolonged dying.

This is precisely where longevity medicine switches to attack mode. It looks for an in-depth understanding of the ageing and degeneration processes in the body. It defines this accumulation of cellular damage and physical loss of function due to advancing age as a disease in its own right and then looks for ways to cure the deadly disease called death. If this scientific paradigm shift finds full political and social acceptance, the research and development game will change radically on a legal and economic level.

Because today, ageing and death are not legally considered diseases but consequences of a wide range of age-related diseases, the US and European drug authorities do not even approve drugs against ageing and death. Even if there were white, yellow, or green pills from our mind game, physicians would not be allowed to prescribe them, and health insurance companies would not be allowed to pay for them. Because of this, pharmaceutical companies have no direct incentive to invest in developing longevity therapeutics. For this reason, for example, findings from basic research on the cell ageing process have until now had difficulties bridging the so-called valley of death of innovation. That means science usually develops state-funded ideas for a medical solution. At some point, the market would have to take over and finance the development of a drug or therapy. But this was and is too risky for the classic market players – the large pharmaceutical companies with corporate roots in the nineteenth and twentieth centuries.

Others are more impatient and less risk-averse. These others are, surprisingly, often men in the second half of their lives who have become incredibly rich through information technology and digital platforms in the first half of their lives and are usually not known to suffer from low self-esteem. Jeff Bezos, co-founder of Amazon, has backed Altos Labs, a company exploring cellular reprogramming to restore aged cells to a youthful state. Google co-founder Larry Page has supported Calico, an Alphabet subsidiary focused on understanding age-related molecular pathways and developing longevity therapeutics. Peter Thiel, ever the contrarian, has channelled millions into Unity Biotechnology, which targets senescent cells – dysfunctional cells that accumulate with age and drive inflammation. Meanwhile, OpenAI CEO Sam Altman has placed a major bet on Retro Biosciences, which aims to extend human lifespan by 10 years through cellular rejuvenation, autophagy enhancement, and blood plasma-based therapies.

Mark Zuckerberg and Priscilla Chan, through the Chan Zuckerberg Initiative, have pledged billions to fight age-related diseases by funding advanced biomedical research in cell ageing and regenerative medicine. Even Vitalik Buterin, the shy European Ethereum co-founder, has invested in SENS Research Foundation, an organization dedicated to reversing ageing at the molecular level. Among the usual suspects, only long-time philanthropist Bill Gates seems to have different priorities. Asked about immortality research on Reddit, he replied: 'It seems pretty egocentric while we still have malaria and TB for rich people to fund things so they can live longer. It would be nice to live longer though I admit'.

Gates aside, tech billionaires' attitude towards longevity medicine unsurprisingly mirrors very much Silicon Valley's digital ethos: moonshot thinking, rapid iteration, and a willingness to challenge scientific dogma. Whether their investments will translate into tangible life-extending therapies within the investors' lifetimes remains uncertain, to say the least. The longevity field has seen its share of hype cycles, where expectations outpace reality. Sceptical physicians, often highly competent, usually consider the promises of longevity researchers and founders to be completely exaggerated. But venture capitalists with a lot of biomedical expertise are betting ever higher sums on scenarios 1 and 2 becoming a reality in their lifetime. Quite a few also believe in the realization of scenario 3.

Chapter 2 of this book highlights who wants to bring about the end of ageing with whose money and what approaches and methods. Spoiler alert: very likely, neither you nor I nor the scientists working on life extension therapies will truly deliver on its bold promises. Even if we had a fully functional anti-ageing therapy today – one that could extend human lifespan by, say, 50 per cent – we would still need to wait at least fifty years to prove that it actually works. Unlike conventional medicine, where the effects of a drug or treatment can often be measured in weeks, months, or a few years, longevity therapies only reveal their true success over an entire human lifetime. Clinical trials, even accelerated ones, cannot fully account for the complex biological and environmental interactions that unfold over decades. The only way to confirm that a therapy prevents ageing in the long run is to observe a population receiving the treatment and compare their lifespan to untreated individuals – a process that inherently spans multiple generations.

This challenge becomes even more daunting if longevity therapies only work when applied at a younger age. If an intervention proves most effective when administered to people in their 20s or 30s, which seems likely, we will have to wait 100 to 125 years to gather definitive evidence that it has truly extended human life expectancy.

The third chapter deals with the question of what a long, extremely long, or theoretically even infinite life could mean for each of us from an individual point of view. Would the groundhog greet us daily and bore us to death in constant loops of repetition? After all, we would have seen and experienced everything multiple times. And perhaps the American writer Susanne Ertz would be right with her laconic remark: Millions long for eternal life. However, they do not even know what to do with themselves on a rainy Sunday afternoon.

Or would longevity finally give us a chance to experience much more than in today's far-too-short lives? Could we remain curious for several centuries, and could we reinvent ourselves again and again, both professionally and personally? What would longevity mean for our friendships, marriages, and relationships with our parents and children? Would suicide no longer be an act of selfishness, peer pressure, or confusion, as the sociologist Émile Durkheim described in his paper *Le suicide* (1897, Eng. *The Suicide*), but the unspectacular default attitude of the long-living towards life? Maybe we could travel to the moon or Mars. Meanwhile, one thing is for sure: here on Earth, the long lives of individuals would force us to renegotiate questions of justice and make significant social changes. This is what the fourth chapter of this book is about.

Let's start with something simple: our pension systems and schemes – public and private – are already on shaky ground today. But how could they cope if life expectancy continues to grow as linearly as it has for the past 150 years? And how should these systems deal economically and organizationally with medical breakthroughs in longevity medicine?

The problem of overpopulation is much more complex. If no one ever dies and everyone continues to live, the global population could exceed 20 billion within a few decades. Wouldn't the logical consequence be that we must ban children, as some well-known sponsors of longevity propose in smaller circles but do not say openly to a broader public?

But this is only the beginning of the problems: Longevity therapies will likely be very costly when introduced. Who can afford them? Will only those internet-platform billionaires who provide venture capital for biotech start-ups have access to progress today? Or would only people in wealthy societies in the northern hemisphere receive free longevity on prescription, while the global South would end up empty-handed?

And tied back to the question of overpopulation: Will only those who opt for longevity interventions or therapies be subject to a (partial) reproductive ban, as the American philosopher John K. Davis, among others, demands? Regulation for longevity will definitely have a substantial impact on lifestyle. Who enforces the ban on children, and what happens to children born 'illegally'? Is a long life without children or a society with few children even desirable? And besides: How innovative and changeable can societies with very many old and very few young people be? Gerontocracy could put humanity in a state of development paralysis.

But here, too, we can design desirable future scenarios. Would many people be willing to act more responsibly today if they knew that they, not only their descendants, would feel the consequences of irresponsible actions first-hand? Or could longevity even allow later generations to set off for exoplanets in other solar systems? With spacecraft propulsion technology available today, the flight there theoretically would take 100,000 years, as Harvard astronomer Avi Loeb calculates. In the future, this should hopefully be much faster.

Of course, this essay cannot give conclusive answers to all these questions. This book aims to shed light on what would be possible and necessary if the premises of scenarios 1 and 2 become a reality in our lifetime or within a few generations. It doesn't just make sense because the probability that these scenarios can occur increases noticeably. We should prepare ourselves in good time for a future with many long-living people because medical tipping points can possibly be quickly reached. More importantly, however, when we design longevity scenarios, we automatically deal with the question of what ageing means to us individually and collectively today. How do we remain curious in later phases of life? How can people use their productivity economically beyond the sixth or seventh life decade? And are we sufficiently sensitized to ageism?

Medicine should enter attack mode through biotechnology. And it is high time to work purposefully and with great effort towards medical breakthroughs because the medical progress of recent decades has not stopped ageing but prolonged dying.

In September 2022, my mother passed away. That was 10 years after her diagnosis of 'Alzheimer's'. It would be a blessing if biotechnology would spare everyone on this Earth – regardless of whether in 30, 50, or 100 years – a similar fate at the end of their life. It would be a blessing if most of us lived healthy and joyful lives for a long time and then passed away quickly. That is surprisingly often the case with the statistical outliers of our species, meaning those who live to be 110 years and older. Herein may lie the most incredible opportunity of longevity medicine.

The above-mentioned (and self-proclaimed) 'Prophet of Longevity', Aubrey de Grey, claims that the first man to live to be a thousand years old has already been born. That's marketing bullshit in the battle for attention. Even if it were possible to completely stop the cell ageing process of the body or even reverse it in specific cells, our brain would still have to remain functional for 1,000 years and free up new storage capacities for new memories. From a medical point of view, it is entirely unclear whether and how this could succeed. Nevertheless, I think it is exciting and sensible to simultaneously consider the extreme scenario with the green pill. This is also, or especially, true if we conclude that immortality would not be a gain for the individual – and certainly not for the human species.

CHAPTER 2

HOW COULD MOLECULAR BIOLOGY AND BIOTECHNOLOGY ACHIEVE MEDICAL BREAKTHROUGHS?

In a creepy-funny scene from the HBO series *Silicon Valley*, a young start-up founder pitches a business idea to the story's anti-hero, venture capitalist Gavin Belson. The founder confidently explains the great opportunities on a graph with an exponential growth curve when another young, handsome man enters the room with a medical device. He sits down next to Belson and couples his own and Belson's basilic veins with tubes to a pump. The irritated founder asks if everything is okay health-wise. On the other hand, investor Belson is irritated that the founder has probably never heard of 'parabiosis'. 'Regularly getting fresh blood from a young, physically fit person can considerably postpone ageing', explains the antihero and introduces the young blood donor: 'This is Brice, my transfusion associate'. The founder should now please continue with his pitch. Apparently, a venture capitalist doesn't have much time, even if he regularly gets rejuvenating live-cell treatments with donor blood.

The villain character Gavin Belson is reminiscent of a mixture of Google founder Sergey Brin, Amazon founder Jeff Bezos, and Facebook investor Peter Thiel. Of course, the scene is satirically exaggerated. But as is often the case with good satire, the evil fun refers to actual circumstances. In this case, two issues are important:

First, parabiosis actually and verifiably leads to physical and cognitive rejuvenation – though not in humans but in mice and rats. The technology is by no means new. As early as the nineteenth century, researchers sutured rodents into Siamese twins, connecting their bloodstreams. In the 1950s, a research team at Cornell University showed that the bone density of an old rat increased again when its bloodstream was forcibly merged with a young rat. The older animal experienced a reversal in osteoporosis. On the other hand, the younger rat aged faster until both met halfway in terms of age. The Cornell results sparked worldwide curiosity. Physicians have now developed numerous similar experiments in Europe and Japan. In the 1970s, it became scientifically certain that parabiosis can significantly prolong the life of laboratory animals overall.

In Germany, parabiosis experiments have been banned since 1987. In the United States and Asia, research has continued investigating the microbiological causes of the rejuvenation effects. Today, we know that young blood in old mice reactivates 'sleeping' stem cells. They begin to divide again and then produce fresh tissue. In the meantime, it is considered scientifically well-established that young blood increases the number of brain cells in old laboratory mice. No one knows exactly why and what this might mean for humans. Until now, we assumed that cells in the brain could not divide and that we would have to make do with the basic equipment from birth for a lifetime. If this assumption is wrong, findings from parabiosis could not only open up new avenues for longevity research but also advance the development of Alzheimer's drugs, for example, based on blood plasma.

Second, the satire about transfusion profiteer Gavin Belson and his young 'transfusion associate', Brice, hits a nerve because the internet money elite of the American West Coast is highly interested in life extension techniques. As mentioned in the last chapter, Sergey Brin, Jeff Bezos, Peter Thiel, Sam Altman, and Oracle founder Larry Ellison have invested in longevity studies and start-ups. Some Russian oligarchs are also active. It is impossible to empirically prove whether their drive comes from a personal desire for infinite life – perhaps the last unfulfillable wish in case of endless wealth – as in the TV series. In their public statements, investors often justify their investments philanthropically. Only people like them, extremely optimistic about technology and financially venturesome, could advance radical medical progress against the disease of death. Everyone could benefit from this. Of course, one motivation does not exclude the other. It is verifiably certain that the sums that risk investors invest in longevity ventures have risen sharply in recent years.

Who Pays the Research Bill?

In January 2022, Altos Labs went down in economic history as the best-funded start-up with three billion US dollars in seed capital. The company is led by cell biologist Richard D. Klausner, who previously headed the American National Cancer Institute with 5,000 employees. Early investors include Russian-Israeli tech investor Yuri Milner and probably Jeff Bezos, who is keeping a low profile regarding his longevity investments. The Supervisory Board includes three Nobel Prize winners: Jennifer Doudna, Frances Arnold Hamilton, and David Baltimore.

In doing so, Altos Labs is undertaking the latest major attempt to bring together digital tech entrepreneurs and leading biotechnologists. In 2013, Google founded its subsidiary California Life Company, Calico for short, and provided it with around 850 million US dollars in capital in the following years.

Also in 2013, biotechnologist Craig Venter, known for his work on gene sequencing, and former Google executive Peter Diamandis founded Human Longevity Inc., based in San Diego. They also quickly raised around $300 million and formed strategic research partnerships with major pharmaceutical companies such as Celgene and AstraZeneca.

In recent years, various non-profit organizations have also managed to raise hundreds of millions of dollars in private capital for research on ageing and then distributed these funds to public or semi-public anti-ageing research teams. One of the best-known is the SENS Research Foundation, which Aubrey de Grey founded in 2009. (de Grey had to leave the board in 2021 over allegations of sexual harassment.) A crucial donor of the SENS Foundation was the Karlsruhe co-founder of Web.de, Michael Greve. In the summer of the same year, he announced that he would invest 300 million euros in 'rejuvenation start-ups' through his investment company Kizoo Technology Ventures. Above all, he would invest in young companies with radical approaches that want to stop the cell ageing process and reverse it. The Israeli-American ageing researcher Nir Barzilai, known for his studies with very old people, so-called centenarians, reports on crypto millionaires under 30 who support his research with millions of dollars, partly as donations without immediate, fixed returns.

In 2021, OpenAI's Sam Altman joined the club of tech entrepreneurs investing in life extension. He poured 180 million dollars into Retro Biosciences. The start-up was founded by

Joe Betts-LaCroix, a Silicon Valley veteran known for building the smallest Windows PC, who has since been involved in various biotech ventures. Betts-LaCroix also founded the Health Extension Foundation, focusing on extending healthy human lifespans. His co-founding scientific lead at Retro Biosciences is Sheng Ding, a prominent scientist in the field of chemical biology and stem cell research. He has made significant contributions to the understanding of cellular reprogramming and regenerative medicine. Accordingly, Retro Biosciences aims to increase healthy human lifespan by 10 years through developing therapies that target the cellular drivers of ageing. As of January 2025, Retro Biosciences has raised an additional $1 billion to advance its mission of extending human lifespan.

Chances seem to be good, as investment in longevity medicine continues to grow. The sector is now firmly on the radar of venture capital funds. Several new longevity-focused venture funds have emerged, including Cambrian BioPharma and Apollo Health Ventures, both of which are structuring portfolios of longevity-focused biotech companies. Investors such as Peter Thiel, Christian Angermayer, and Laura Deming's Longevity Fund have also increased their stakes in longevity biotech.

As venture capital continues to push forward with private funding, public research institutions have become more adaptive. Both in the United States and Europe, government-backed initiatives now co-fund longevity research, especially where overlaps exist with combating age-related diseases such as cancer, dementia, and diabetes. The hope is to create synergy where venture capital catalyses fundamental research, which in turn attracts further private funding, driving longevity medicine closer to mainstream clinical applications.

This said, it is also obvious that the biggest hopes of longevity investment enthusiasts have not materialized yet. In 2022, Human Longevity Inc. had announced an IPO, which would have been the first in the industry. It has been postponed ever since. Seasoned mainstream scientists often remain sceptical, pointing to a long history of announced 'medical breakthroughs' that have led to nothing neither for patients with age-related diseases nor postponing death overall. The potential return on investment in longevity therapy may be almost infinite, hence any quick pay-off seems more than unlikely. Maybe it is this chasm that attracts the flock of chancers and even charlatans since medieval alchemists. They come in a variety of colours nowadays.

Dubious, high-risk approaches to speed up the death of death have recently spurned at the intersections of the crypto bro community, self-experimental biohackers, and political libertarians defying 'overregulation'. One of the most prominent figures in this scene is Bryan Johnson. The tech entrepreneur, author, and longevity social media star, born in 1977, attracted worldwide attention a few years ago when he tried to rejuvenate his own body with the blood plasma of his 17-year-old son. In videos on his YouTube channel and a Netflix documentary, Johnson's fans and critics can follow how he tries to turn back his biological clock using experimental rejuvenation methods. Johnson calls it 'Project Blueprint' and seems to feel comfortable in his multiple roles of guru, trailblazer, and guinea pig. One of his settings for these experiments is 'Próspera', a low-regulation, low-tax free trade zone on the island of Roatan in Honduras. The Honduran government set up this 'free zone' in 2013, primarily to provide the emerging crypto scene with an experimental space for new business models centred around blockchain technology. American libertarians including former Coinbase CTO Balaji Srinivasan, star investor Marc Andreesen, and, of course, Peter Thiel have financially backed the project. Individuals can apply for 'e-residency', which allows them to register businesses in Próspera and benefit from the local tax and regulatory structure. Bitcoin is the official currency in Próspera. Hence, lean regulation does not only apply to financial services.

A number of biotech start-ups have also set up shop there, mostly financed with crypto millions. Together, they form Vitalia Longevity City, where one can find offers to upgrade one's body into a cyborg, but also to undergo stem cell therapies that are not approved by the American or European regulatory authorities – the U.S. Food and Drug Administration (FDA) and the European Medicines Agency (EMA). The ideological overlaps between crypto and experimental rejuvenation medicine are obvious. The consensus in Próspera is that over-regulation hinders technical progress, and there is hardly any other industry that is as over-regulated as pharmaceuticals. This attitude has, in turn, attracted companies such as Minicircle to Próspera. The start-up administers gene therapy which targets a protein called follistatin to rapidly build muscles. Bryan Johnson is its most prominent customer. The rudimentary studies that Minicircle has published on this therapy have caused renowned scientists to shake their heads.

At the same time, the success of influencers such as Bryan Johnson and the existence of virtually lawless longevity experimentation centres such as Vitalia Longevity City are just another sign that no price seems too high for many people to pay to beat death, even if that price is their own health. The radical offence mode of longevity biohackers is often considered radically irresponsible by mainstream scientists. That doesn't mean that radical (or irresponsible) innovators don't rely on the same mainstream research that might open the doors to slow down or even reverse the process of ageing. Longevity therapy is hard to come by. But scientific knowledge about the biomolecular process of ageing has advanced tremendously in the last two decades.

What Happens Biologically in the Body When We Age?

Simply put, ageing is a gradual process of biological decline, affecting every cell, tissue, and organ in the body. Over time, damage accumulates, cellular repair mechanisms weaken, and physiological functions deteriorate, increasing susceptibility to disease and eventually leading to death. While ageing was once considered an inevitable and poorly understood phenomenon, scientific advances over the past decades have provided deeper insights into its underlying mechanisms. A breakthrough came in 2013, when the Spanish biologist Carlos López-Otín and four colleagues published their seminal paper outlining nine hallmarks of ageing – a framework identifying the key molecular and cellular processes driving biological ageing. This model became widely accepted in longevity research and served around the globe as a foundation for developing potential anti-ageing therapies.

In 2023, López-Otín and his team expanded this framework to 12 hallmarks, incorporating recent discoveries. Some longevity experts now refer to these 12 hallmarks as the 'dirty dozen of ageing', as they highlight the interconnected biological failures that contribute to age-related decline. These hallmarks provide a structured way to analyse how and why we age at the molecular and cellular levels.

For all who want to dig a little bit deeper into the biomedical causes of ageing and age-related diseases, here is a short overview.

AGEING'S DIRTY DOZEN

Primary

Damage to fundamental cell components: DNA, chromosomes, proteome, and organelles.

1. Genomic Instability

Our DNA is constantly exposed to damage from environmental factors like radiation, toxins, and metabolic by-products. While cells have repair mechanisms, these become less efficient over time, leading to mutations, chromosomal abnormalities, and mitochondrial dysfunction, all of which contribute to ageing because they, simply put, stop genes from working the way they should.

2. Telomere Attrition

Telomeres are protective caps at the ends of chromosomes that shorten with each cell division. When telomeres become critically short, cells enter a state of senescence or die. This process is one of the key factors in tissue deterioration and ageing-related diseases because it stymies cell division.

3. Epigenetic Alterations

Ageing leads to changes in the way genes are expressed, even without alterations to the DNA sequence itself. These epigenetic changes can switch off beneficial genes or activate harmful ones, contributing to cellular dysfunction, inflammation, and disease. In short, as markers on chromosomes change, cells don't know any more what genes they should use.

4. Loss of Proteostasis

Cells need to maintain a balanced system of protein production, folding, and degradation. As we age, this system becomes impaired. Cells produce proteins in non-functional forms and wrong numbers, leading to the accumulation of misfolded and damaged proteins, which contribute to neurodegenerative diseases like Alzheimer's and Parkinson's.

5. Disabled Autophagy

Autophagy is the body's cellular recycling system, clearing damaged proteins and organelles. In ageing, autophagy declines and can no longer break down components, leading to toxic buildup, mitochondrial dysfunction, inflammation, and neurodegeneration, accelerating age-related diseases and cellular decline.

Antagonistic

Mechanisms compensating for damage done by malfunctioning primary mechanisms.

6. Deregulated Nutrient Sensing

Cells rely on nutrient-sensing pathways, such as insulin signalling and mTOR, to regulate metabolism. As we age, these pathways become dysregulated. The cell's energy metabolism suffers, contributing to metabolic disorders like diabetes and obesity, which accelerate ageing.

7. Mitochondrial Dysfunction

Mitochondria, the energy powerhouses of the cell, become less efficient with age. This leads to lower energy production and increased oxidative stress, damaging cells and contributing to age-related diseases.

8. Cellular Senescence

Some cells lose their ability to divide and function properly, entering a state known as senescence. These 'zombie cells' secrete harmful molecules that cause inflammation and tissue degradation, accelerating ageing.

Integrative

Impaired or damaging responses to change.

9. Stem Cell Exhaustion

Stem cells are responsible for regenerating tissues, but their number and function decline with age. They divide less and reproduce fewer new cells. This results in slower healing, reduced immune function, and increased frailty.

10. Altered Intercellular Communication

Ageing disrupts communication between cells. Cells coordinate much less, leading to chronic inflammation and a weakened ability to respond to stress and injury. This contributes to multiple age-related diseases, including cardiovascular conditions.

11.   Chronic Inflammation (Inflammaging)

The body unnecessarily sends out messages calling for an inflammatory response.

Low-grade, persistent inflammation is a key driver of ageing. It is caused by immune system dysfunction, senescent cells, and metabolic imbalances, increasing the risk of cancer, heart disease, and neurodegeneration.

12.   Dysbiosis (Microbiome Imbalance)

The gut microbiome, essential for digestion and immunity, changes unfavourably with age. This imbalance leads to increased inflammation, metabolic disorders, and a weakened immune response.

Understanding these hallmarks of ageing is key for all attempts to develop strategies or therapies to expand humans' average healthspan or eventually break the lifetime glass ceiling of 120 or so years. This applies to relatively simple countermeasures like a change in diet or frequent exposure to cold or weightlifting in older age, as practised by many who subscribe to the trend of longevity lifestyles. But a deep knowledge is even more crucial to advance with highly sophisticated interventions in human metabolism or genetic code.

Which Longevity Approaches Promise Success?

Fasting, exposure to cold, exercise

Suppose you significantly reduce the calories of nematodes, mice, rats, fish, and rhesus monkeys and at the same time keep the nutrients in their diet high. In that case, their lifespan is extended, and they continue to live healthily. In mice, this extends their lifespan by around 40 per cent. Among longevity devotees, diets with radical calorie restriction (so-called CR diets) and high nutrient supply are all the rage, especially in the United States. Meaningful long-term studies with humans are not yet available, which is the nature of things. The studies only started a few years ago, and people would become quite old before reliable data on actual success can be available.

To make matters worse, CR diets are very complex regarding purchase and preparation, and those fasting long-term are constantly hungry, which leads to high dropout rates. However, interim results with a smaller number of subjects indicate that the diet achieves the desired effects, at least for cardiovascular diseases. According to a study by the Washington School of Medicine, those who consistently live according to the CR diet have cardiac values of people 20 years younger who eat an average healthy diet. Intermittent fasting, cold exposure, and intense workout sessions can also trigger rejuvenating effects. The microbiological reason seems to be the same as for CR.

Fasting, cold exposure, and exercise can naturally increase so-called NAD^+ levels. When fasting, the body shifts into a repair mode, conserving and recycling NAD^+ while improving mitochondrial function. Cold exposure activates brown fat, which burns energy to generate heat, increasing NAD^+ production in the process. Physical exertion, especially intense exercise, pushes muscles to demand more energy, prompting the body to produce additional NAD^+ to fuel metabolism and repair cells. These natural stressors help maintain cellular function, slow ageing, and promote overall health by supporting efficient energy use and resilience.

NAD^+, in turn, is the prerequisite for the so-called sirtuins to do their job well. Sirtuins belong to epigenetic regulators. These 'longevity genes' assign cells their respective tasks when they arise or divide in the body. The younger the body, the smoother this process works. In old age, this control function of the sirtuins gradually decreases because they perform a second important task. The second job of the 'longevity genes' is to be the cells' fire department and technical relief organization. They are always used where viral or bacterial fires need to be extinguished, or DNA needs repairing. The older we get, the more frequently the sirtuins are in disaster response, and the less often they can ensure that our cells renew themselves like those of a child or adolescent.

Stimulating cell functions with rapamycin and metformin

Conversely, all this means that those who manage to keep the production of NAD^+ in the cells permanently high age more slowly. However, most people are reluctant to starve and freeze. Unfortunately, physical exertion is exhausting. Who can and wants to keep this up for a lifetime? In addition, the correct dosage is difficult with all three natural methods. Most people would most likely only consider drugs to achieve the same effect. Promising candidates for this are the active ingredients rapamycin, obtained from a fungus-inhibiting bacterium from the Easter Island Rapa Nui and the relatively cheap diabetes drug metformin. Both are NAD^+ stimulators and seem to have a positive effect on the so-called TOR gene. TOR also takes over repair work in the cells if it does not have to satisfy its primary task of organizing the metabolism in case of high food intake.

In fruit flies and mice, rapamycin and metformin prolong the so-called healthspan – the phase of our lives in which we are healthy – as well as lifespan. That this is also the case in humans seems likely but is not yet sufficiently proven. The long-term studies are too short here, too, so the interim results are not very meaningful. Similar to NAD^+ and TOR stimulation, studies aim to better regulate the so-called insulin growth factor (IGF) in old age. The medical hypothesis here is: At high levels of IGF, cells in organisms tend to grow. At low levels, they require maintenance and repair. However, the search in connection with IGF-active ingredients has only just begun.

Research approaches of the protein class of chaperones are also young. These support newly formed proteins in cells during folding and shield them from coming into contact with harmful proteins and then tangling up into damaging protein clusters. Hence the name: Chaperone, which means 'lady of decency'.

Researchers are paying more and more attention to the enzymatic processes with the cells' waste disposal and recycling functions. In the so-called lysis, impaired proteins are first crushed. Subsequently, they are transported out of the cells, and the precious material is recycled. Evolution has developed these complex cellular processes extremely cleverly and efficiently. Unfortunately, they function worse and worse with increasing age – presumably precisely because of their high complexity. The goal is clear: If we succeed in keeping the cells' waste disposal and recycling stable for longer, we will age more slowly. There is still a long way to go for all the approaches mentioned here.

Senolytics and telomerase

Among the best-known and most promising approaches in longevity research are senolytics and telomerase. Senotherapy is also about a waste disposal function – not within the cell, but of senescent cells, also called zombie cells. The undead among the cell tissue no longer divide and fulfil their programmed functions. However, senescent cells do not die off and thus make way for the next cell generation. Instead, their metabolism continues to run at full speed. This way, they block the entire renewal process. Zombie cells likely play an important role in dementia. An essential key against age-related diseases of the brain could lie in killing the zombies and transporting them out. An even more elegant biomedical method would be not to let them develop in the first place but to make cells much more durable from the outset, which is the telomerase approach.

The ends of our DNA strands are called telomeres. They prevent the strands of our DNA from fraying and work similarly to the small plastic protective caps at the ends of shoelaces. With each cell division, the telomeres shorten. At some point, they become too short. In the best-case scenario, the cell kills itself by apoptosis through enzymes. In the worst-case scenario, it mutates into a zombie cell. The human body has developed a natural defence mechanism against telomere shortening: the enzyme telomerase can lengthen telomeres in continuously dividing cells such as germ cells, stem cells, and specific immune cells. Unfortunately, an old body does not produce enough of this enzyme. Here, the research question is: How can telomerase be produced sufficiently so that old cells continue to divide?

Stem cell therapy and artificial organs

In senolytics and telomerase, science is progressing slowly but steadily. It is difficult to predict when the first anti-ageing products will be approved. Their effect could be considerable but probably not as effective as the most powerful levers of longevity medicine from today's perspective. These include stem cell therapy, artificial organs, and genome editing.

Stem cells are all-rounders. They produce specialists among cells. An embryo initially consists exclusively of (so-called pluripotent) stem cells. They build the body in its hardly comprehensible complexity with active division and function assignment to cells such as blood, skin, or kidney cells. In the growth phase of childhood and adolescence, stem cells are at their peak. But even as adults, we still have plenty of them. They then further renew the tissues and organs with new specialist cells. However, after the peak of the reproductive phase, starting in the fourth decade of life, the ability of stem cells decreases. The number of stem cells also decreases continuously.

To this day, science has only scratched the surface of understanding how exactly stem cell degradation and signs of ageing are causally related. Accordingly, science is uncertain about recommending therapeutic approaches. Stem cell therapies with spinal cord donor cells for blood cancer could provide important information. Functional stem cells from an (often younger) donor allow blood cancer patients to overcome death by replacing the blood cell-producing stem cells that have been knocked out of control by cancer.

Another approach leads outside the body: thanks to stem cells, mass-produced organs for every ageing person could be grown in the laboratory. Heart and kidney, eye and blood vessel: all of them could be available in the just-in-time spare parts warehouse and, with regular maintenance, be replaced fully automatically by surgical robots in the distant future.

However, a significant challenge for longevity research in stem cell therapies is to avoid relying on donor cells. Suitable donors are hard to find, and because of the complicated removal of cells, you can hardly demand this because of ethical reasons. Therefore, the aim is to clone fully functional stem cells from one's own body or to reprogramme other cells into pluripotent all-rounders.

The Japanese stem cell researcher Shin'ya Yamanaka laid the scientific foundation for this in 2006. In mouse cells, he modified four so-called transcription factors – proteins that switch off certain sections of the DNA. In turn, the four Yamanaka factors suffice to return differentiated mouse body cells and the genetic information in their nuclei to the state of embryonic stem cells. For this finding, he received the Nobel Prize in Medicine in 2012. However, the approach is not yet sufficiently developed for use against general ageing in humans.

Artificially generated pluripotent stem cells have the unpleasant effect of causing cancerous tumours, so-called teratomas. Biomedicine will likely get a grip on the undesirable side effects of cell reprogramming. So the question is when rather than if it will succeed. The rapid progress in biotechnology tools, such as ever-better gene shears, gives genetic engineers cause for optimism. At this point, we would be at the most far-reaching approaches of longevity research: direct interventions in human DNA.

Gene editing

Today, geneticists know several dozen genes that influence the ageing process, which we humans share with many animals, yeast, and other multicellular organisms. In many experiments, it has been possible to manipulate these ageing genes (and their interactions) in gene regulation networks (GRN) so that yeast cultures, worms, fruit flies, and rodents age healthier and live longer. The aim has always been to eliminate genetically coded ageing functions and to strengthen renewal or repair mechanisms already established by nature. Of course, both must be possible without serious side effects that can bring us closer to death again, making things even more difficult.

The alteration of gene function can occur through drugs introduced into the cells, such as by introducing mRNA. Some ageing-relevant active ingredients of these gene therapies are already in clinical trials in the hope that they will be approved for cancer therapy and against diabetes. We can expect significant progress in the coming years. However, it will take a few decades to know precisely what effects they actually have on ageing. Even more promising are tools such as the gene shears CRISPR, with which biotechnologists can cut and change DNA in a targeted manner.

Jennifer Doudna and Emmanuelle Charpentier received the Nobel Prize in Chemistry in 2020 for developing the CRISPR-Cas9 method. The gene shears available today work with enzymes (the Cas) with which individual DNA sequences can be removed from the entire strand in a targeted way and replaced. Animal experiments give reason to hope that resounding therapeutic successes in many diseases, from cancer to haemophilia and malaria to sickle cell and Huntington's disease, could be achieved with gene editing. CRISPR has simplified gene editing so that biohackers can (and do) conduct self-experiments, for example, to improve their night vision with cat genes. So far, the CRISPR gene shears, figuratively speaking, probably have the precision of coarse paper scissors. No one knows what will be possible with the next generations of genetic modification methods with much higher precision and growing knowledge of genetics. Gene editing – combined with bioinformatics to unlock the secrets of molecular biological processes through mass data – is the biggest miracle bag of longevity research.

There may be biotechnological innovations in this miracle bag that can significantly shift the age limit in one fell swoop. But perhaps much less will come of it than genetic engineers and synthetic biologists loudly promise when looking for capital.

Nanobots, mind-upload, cryonics

Futurists and transhumanists like Ray Kurzweil think conceptually bigger in the game of eternal life – and technically somewhat smaller. They predict (or hope) that in the indeterminate future, nanobots could whizz through our bodies – at the push of a button from the physician or on the advice of an algorithm – and control those organs where maintenance work is due or acute intervention is necessary.

If future generations of physicians fail in significantly shifting the biological age limit, computer scientists and AI scientists may be driving considerable leaps in innovation instead. According to the cyborg community, our descendants could upload their consciousness (or soul?) to a computer network in the future. We could then continue to live forever in cyberspace without biological bodies.

Among the colourful array of revolutionary technology utopians, we also encounter cryonicists. As medical progress may not come as fast as they have wished for, cryonicists aim to bridge time into a more innovative future. After death, they preserve their bodies in liquid nitrogen at minus 196 degrees Celsius and hope that some longevity method will eventually become a medical reality. The fact that physicians will be able to bring frozen people back to life in the future is a prerequisite for them. At first glance, this bet on medical progress may not be so bad, especially since offers for freezing in the United States start at $30,000. It gets much cheaper if you only freeze your head or brain. Several thousand people have already been put into nitrogen after dying or arranged it for the time of their death. But not everything runs smoothly: since the 1970s, some cryonics companies have gone bankrupt. In these incidents, the dead customers were buried per their contract. Of course, the frozen bet can only work if the backup batteries don't fail when called upon over the next 300 years.

It may be inappropriate to dismiss futuristic methods as complete nonsense. Even in these cases, of course, we cannot know what humanity will know and be able to do in a hundred or a thousand years. We know, however, that we do not yet know how such breakthroughs could become technically possible. Despite all the scientific uncertainty and necessary scepticism about the marketing talk, this no longer applies to the described molecular biological and genetic advances in longevity medicine.

Ageing in 2145

With all this promising research, scenarios in which many people are significantly older than Jeanne Calment are 'plausible' from today's perspective. Scenario research understands this to mean that if current data and trends continue, 'plausible' scenarios can actually become a reality. However, we cannot calculate a specific probability of occurrence for this to happen.

The Frenchwoman Jeanne Calment is the only person who was verifiably over 120 years old. (Some cast doubts about her being much younger due to an identity swap by her daughter, which went viral in 2018, have been convincingly dismissed by several thorough investigations by various scientists.) Her life and lifestyle at the highest age remain uncontestably unique.

Calment was still riding a bicycle when she was over 100 years old. It was not until she was 110 that she moved into a nursing home. At the age of 118, she gave up smoking, not for health reasons, but because she could no longer light her cigarettes herself. Her independence was too important to her to depend on others when smoking. Chocolate and port wine continued to be a welcome treat.

Jeanne Calment was born in Arles on 21 February 1875. She died in 1997 at the age of 122 years and 164 days. In 1875, her countryman Louis Pasteur discovered that germs transmit diseases. At the time, no one knew that there was such a thing as genes that pass on genetic information. When Calment was a child, science discovered X-rays. Throughout her life, chemists, biologists, physicians, and pharmacologists developed insulin and penicillin, chemotherapy for cancer, vaccinations for almost all childhood diseases, dialysis, and statins. When Jeanne Calment died on 4 August 1997, as the oldest person ever, we had almost decoded the human genome.

A child born today as I write this, who lived as long as Calment, would live to see the year 2145. This child probably has some, perhaps many, decades of healthy life ahead of him or her. In the next two chapters, we'll ask, what personal challenges might arise in the face of extreme longevity compared to our lives today? And what could this mean for societies in which many people live as old as giant tortoises, Greenland sharks – or even older?

CHAPTER 3

WOULD A LONG LIFE BE
DEADLY BORING?

David William Goodall was born in North London just before World War I began. In 1935, at 21, he received his Bachelor of Science degree from the prestigious Imperial College. At the outbreak of World War II, the Royal Navy called him in for a medical examination. Despite his medical fitness, the doctoral botany student was not drafted for military service. His research was considered extremely important given the food scarcity, also and especially for British agriculture.

In 2017, Goodall was a guest on an Australian talk show. The moderator asked him: 'Why do you still go to your office at the university four days a week?' The 103-year-old replied: 'What else am I supposed to do?' Unfortunately, he can no longer go out into the field to do experiments because running in the field is now quite difficult for him. 'I have no choice but to review and publish scientific studies at my desk', said Australia's oldest active scientist. The audience and moderator laughed. At 103, Goodall's sense of humour still worked across generations.

During his seven-decade-long scientific career in England, with professorships in the United States, Africa, and Australia, Goodall published more than a hundred of his studies. In his field, he became known for statistical models for plant communities. Goodall officially retired in 1979. He simply continued to teach and research at the University of Perth in Western Australia. Goodall was spared severe illnesses. At just under 100, the plant researcher was still editor-in-chief of the 30-volume book series *Ecosystems of the World*.

But then one year after the talk show Goodall fell in his apartment and was not found until two days later. His doctors advised him to move to a nursing home. Instead, he flew to Switzerland and ended his life on 10 May 2018, supported by the euthanasia organization Eternal Spirit. On the eve of his assisted suicide, he gave an interview in Basel: he demanded that active euthanasia finally be legalized in Australia. And he emphasized: 'I am happy to end a happy life'.

When Souls Age

David Goodall was allowed to live life (with small sacrifices and, of course, without a white miracle pill) according to the first scenario of our thought experiment. This makes him part of a small minority in two ways: few live to be over 100 years old. And only a few of the very old are still mentally fit, fundamentally optimistic, and in good spirits – without suffering chronic pain. The first major task of longevity medicine is to make such exceptions the norm.

Very old people's lives today are usually even more difficult than young people could imagine. For many seniors, being awake means feeling pain. Many sensory organs function poorly or no longer function at all. Even if the brain is still cognitively efficient, very elderly people often hear, see, smell, and taste badly or not at all. In the worst case, they also experience anxiety and depression.

This is how Ursula Müller-Werdan, director of the Department of Geriatrics and Gerontology at Charité Berlin, describes the lives of many of her patients. Müller-Werdan does not belong to the futurist faction among physicians. But she also considers ageing a disease and assumes that in the coming decades, there will be many more people who will live a long life in relatively good physical and mental condition. 'If you're healthy, you might still have fun at 115', says the Berlin ageing researcher. In turn, she points out that the psychological aspects are often underestimated in discussions about longevity. Or they are completely overlooked out of sheer euphoria about progress in delaying cellular ageing processes.

If medicine succeeds in stopping physical ageing in the coming decades, the problem of ageing of the soul will still have to be solved. Fundamentally, mental ageing is initially decoupled from physical ageing. So, if you want the white pill from the thought experiment, you should consider this: even with good health and material prosperity, it is usually a great challenge to make the time between 80 and 100 meaningful and joyful. Scientists can pursue their passion even with gradually decreasing performance and low external pressure to perform. But how does a smooth transition from gainful employment to fulfilling work in old age succeed for middle school teachers, nurses, or roofers? Even at the age of 115, some people may still be able to pass the time meaningfully. However, for many this would probably have to be socially organized. Social connection is at least as important for mental well-being in old age as in adolescence and midlife, but it is more challenging to arrange. Even if the very elderly are actually still mobile, their openness to new social relationships often decreases.

And then, there is the psychological effect of 'subjective time acceleration'. As even the middle-aged among us know all to well: when we get older, time seems to pass more quickly due to several psychological and neurological factors. One major explanation is the proportional theory, which suggests that as we age, each year becomes a smaller fraction of our total life. For a 10-year-old, a year is 10 per cent of their life, whereas for a 50-year-old, it's only 2 per cent, making it feel much shorter in comparison. Another key factor is neural processing speed. The brain's ability to process new experiences and encode memories slows down over time. In childhood, everything is novel, and the brain actively records new experiences, creating a dense timeline of events. As adults, we experience fewer 'firsts' and rely more on routine, reducing the number of memorable moments. With fewer distinct memories, time appears to have passed more quickly when we look back. Childhood summers lasted forever, while decades in adulthood seem to fly by.

How compressed will time feel for a 150-year-old? How much subjective time gain will an additional year mean for her or him? How much happiness or pleasure will another life decade add for a 300-year-old? An economist with an interest in psychology and longevity medicine might predict that life might become inflationary. Marginal benefits will decrease sharply the older we get, even if we might stay physically and psychologically healthy.

Ursula Müller-Werdan is convinced that scenario 1 can only become a desirable future for an individual if curiosity and interest in others are maintained – ideally for new relationships and perhaps even new love relationships. This is probably possible but certainly not easy. On the other hand, many very old people could make new alliances with each other in such a future. Could this be a key to happily in young bodies? If so, Western cultures might not be best prepared for an age of longevity.

Ageing Alone?

The dominant Western narrative of 'successful ageing' reveals a profound ideological bias that conflates human worth with productivity, economic utility, and individual achievement. This perspective, deeply rooted in a market-driven logic, reduces the potential of extended human life to a series of optimized performances – a relentless mandate to remain economically and personally 'active'. This looks like a perfect cultural trap for a society with many super-centenarians, even if they might be, on average, in good health.

Eastern philosophical traditions might offer a much more helpful conception. In contrast to the Western hyper-individualized model, Eastern perspectives – particularly those from Confucian, Buddhist, and certain Indigenous traditions – conceptualize ageing as a collective and relational process. Here, longevity is not about personal maintenance or continued professional productivity, but about deepening social wisdom, intergenerational knowledge transmission, and community integration.

The 'successful ageing' paradigm, popularized by the US-American gerontologist Robert Butler, paradoxically creates a new form of social pressure. Older individuals are expected to remain entrepreneurial subjects – constantly reinventing themselves, maintaining physical fitness, pursuing new skills, and resisting any perception of decline. This approach instrumentalizes extended life, transforming it into a performance of perpetual self-optimization.

In many Eastern cultures, elders are seen as repositories of collective memory and social knowledge. Their value isn't measured by economic output but by their capacity to maintain social coherence, provide emotional support, and transmit cultural practices. A 150- or 200-year-old individual could be imagined not as a hyper-productive entrepreneur but as a profound social connector – someone who bridges multiple generational experiences and maintains complex social networks.

This perspective suggests that meaningful longevity isn't mainly about individual resilience but about deepening social relationships. Extended life becomes an opportunity for expanded empathy, more nuanced understanding of human complexity, and the cultivation of profound inter-human connections that transcend immediate economic utility. After all, long-living humans would have much more time to deepen their social skills and common understanding. These deep social bonds could then lead to more happiness for them individually and for societies overall, creating a world very different from most future narratives which entail longevity.

The Struldbrug Dystopia

In classic literature, movies, and TV series, longevity has an utterly bad reputation. The long-living are mostly pitiful, often vile characters. Over the decades, Oscar Wilde's *Dorian Grey* becomes increasingly greedy, self-indulgent, and cruel. His sins are inscribed in his image for all to see. Undead and vampires have filled a whole genre of horror books, movies, musicals, and computer games with blood. One can feel sorry for the tragic heroine Emilia Marty in the Czech opera *The Makropulos Affair* when she becomes a guinea pig for her father's alchemical experiments. As an unfortunate femme fatale at 42, she wanders through the centuries with changing names. She manically turns men's heads until she finally concludes at the age of 342: death is better than life. The Flying Dutchman has a similar experience. Sailing forever is unbearable, even when sailing is his greatest passion.

Things are even worse for the immortal Struldbrugs from *Gulliver's Travels*: when Lemuel Gulliver first hears about them on the island of Luggnagg, he initially envies them for their 'limitless possibilities' and 'divine freedom'. However, the island's mortals laugh at Gulliver because he obviously confuses eternal life with eternal youth. The Struldbrugs are subject to a different fate. They age forever and become frail, bored, disagreeable, cynical shadows of themselves. Their actual function quickly becomes clear to Gulliver: the mortals are constantly reminded by the Struldbrugs that they should be grateful for a finite life. Gulliver himself determines: 'I grew heartily ashamed of the pleasing visions I had formed; and thought no tyrant could invent a death into which I would not run with pleasure, from such a life'. And what about the poor 'Highlander'?

Connor MacLeod's immortality forces him to watch everyone he loves grow old and die while he remains unchanged, creating an endless cycle of loss and emotional detachment. This is particularly poignant in his relationship with his first wife Heather, whom he must watch age and die while he remains eternally young. The pain of these accumulated losses leads him to become increasingly guarded about forming deep connections, knowing they will inevitably end in grief.

Even in the, by definition, tech-savvy genre of science fiction, longevity leads surprisingly often to dystopia. A more recent example is the Netflix series *Altered Carbon*, set in the twenty-fourth century. Consciousness can be stored digitally. Therefore, the killing of human bodies is only considered property damage. The affluent class of immortal 'Meths' often and with pleasure kills under these conditions. And the Netflix movie *Paradise* takes the same theme to the ultimate capitalistic dystopian level.

The story unfolds in a near-future society where AEON, a powerful biotech corporation, has developed a revolutionary technology allowing people to transfer years of their lives to others. While this process is marketed as a way to fight ageing and provide financial security, it quickly becomes a tool of exploitation, where the wealthy buy youth from the desperate. To cut a long story short: the rich extend their lives at the expense of the poor, who are coerced into selling their futures for short-term survival. Human lifespan becomes a marketable commodity.

Of course, there are oeuvres in traditional literature and pop culture, shedding positive light on biomedically extended life. Various *Star Trek* storylines depict extended lifespans as a means to achieve greater wisdom, exploration, and cultural enrichment. In Arthur C. Clarke's *Childhood's End*, humanity gradually evolves into a higher state of being under the guidance of an advanced alien race – extended lifespan included. And the visually stunning film *The Fountain* explores themes of immortality through multiple timelines, ultimately suggesting that the quest for longevity can be intertwined with spiritual enlightenment and love rather than fear or suffering. But these are rather exceptions.

Most fiction on longevity is prone to create a top 10 list of downsides:

1. Psychological Isolation – The crushing loneliness of watching all loved ones age and die while remaining unchanged, leading to emotional withdrawal and an inability to form new bonds for fear of inevitable loss.
2. Character Corruption – Extended life gradually erodes morality and empathy. The immortal becomes increasingly detached from humanity, viewing mortals as insignificant and temporary, often developing god complexes or cruel tendencies.
3. Social Inequality – Life extension becomes a tool of class warfare, with the wealthy hoarding longevity technology while the poor age and die normally, creating new and extreme forms of social stratification.

4. Loss of Purpose – Without death providing a natural end point, life loses its urgency and meaning. Immortals struggle with crushing boredom, lack of motivation, and the inability to find purpose in unlimited time.

5. Memory Burden – The weight of accumulated memories and traumas becomes unbearable over centuries, leading to various forms of psychological dysfunction or memory loss as a coping mechanism.

6. Social Stagnation – Long-lived individuals become resistant to change and progress, effectively becoming living fossils unable to adapt to evolving times and holding back societal advancement.

7. Resource Competition – Extended lifespans lead to overpopulation and increased competition for limited resources, often resulting in societal collapse or strict population control measures.

8. Identity Crisis – The difficulty of maintaining a coherent sense of self over centuries of existence, as personalities shift and memories fade or become unreliable.

9. Generational Conflict – Deep tensions between the long-lived and normal-lifespan populations, often leading to violence or societal breakdown as younger generations resist the control of the eternally old.

10. Natural Order Disruption – The suggestion that immortality is fundamentally 'unnatural' and its pursuit inevitably leads to unforeseen negative consequences for both individuals and society.

But why does eternal life so often have such a bad reputation in culture? Are the authors – and we as a society – subject to mental self-restraint true to the principle: since we have not had a chance to become healthy and happy, active and curious 150-year-olds or older, literature and culture concentrate on the advantages of finiteness? Or did French existentialists like Jean-Paul Sartre, Simone de Beauvoir, and Albert Camus leave such a strong impression? And do we gloss over death because we know it will inevitably come? Perhaps religious conditioning still plays a vital role in the defensive attitude of overcoming death, even in secular cultures. With immortality on Earth, the Christian narrative of eternal life would finally become obsolete, thanks to divine salvation. However, the creation of man is a task of God, not a social mission for molecular biologists. The atheistic, that is, the rational-scientific, corresponding idea is that with longevity research, human beings are messing with evolution with such force that the attempt is likely to cause significantly more harm than good. So, should already the attempt be punishable?

Life and Death, Love and Boredom

Longevity enthusiasts are convinced that humanity will immediately overcome its self-limiting mindset if the biotechnological possibility exists to radically prolong life in good health. Everyone will want to swallow the white and yellow pills as soon as they become available. An indication of this could be how difficult it is for people to let go of life, even if they suffer great pain, disabilities, and psychological stress. The longing and sovereign decision for (assisted) suicide, when the time comes, remains the exception, not the rule. When the time comes, most of us agree with the core ideas of the American philosopher Thomas Nagel: death robs us of our existence and, thus, the possibility of further experiences. It takes everything from us, regardless of when it comes and what we might experience after death. For Nagel, this is 'bad'. Accordingly, it is rational to want to continue living as long as possible. We think it is generally better if a person dies at the age of 90 and not already at the age of 10. So why shouldn't it be better to die at 190 than at 90? Life makes sense when the living person considers it to be meaningful. Theoretically, this also applies to eternal life.

The British ethicist Bernard Williams advocates the antithesis to Nagel: death is good. Williams said eternal life must lead to unbearable boredom because we have to go through the same experiences over and over again. Apart from death, there is only one alternative to this problem: to avoid unbearable boredom, we would have to change ourselves so much that we would no longer be ourselves. Longevity would mean a complete change in identity. The 20-year-old Bernard Williams would have nothing in common with the 200- or 2000-year-old except for the body, which is biotechnologically kept young. Eternal life would become a series of independent and separate lives. Sartre put it this way: 'Even if we were immortal, we would remain finite beings'. But then the entire biotechnical effort would be pointless. Either way, nature lines up life after life. Our genes live on in our descendants.

In the discussions after my lectures on longevity, the challenge of 'boredom' almost always leads to arguments, often surprisingly emotional. The majority usually agrees with William's position. Death gives our lives the needed urgency. We do something because we know that we don't have infinite time. We develop deep relationships and experience unforgettable emotional moments that we often feel were made for eternity because we ultimately know that we cannot be with others indefinitely. The already mentioned Queen song 'Who Wants to Live Forever?' ends with:

> Touch my world with your fingertips
> And we can have forever
> And we can love forever
> Forever is our today.

Through love, we experience infinity in the moment. Infinity is our now.

Bernard Williams argues with the logic of the reverse conclusion of the Queen song. An almost inevitable consequence of longevity would be superficiality. If death no longer necessarily ends our lives, so the assumption goes, we would have to die an inner death, a death of inner desolation. What makes matters worse is the phenomenon of subjectively accelerating time. In childhood, a year seems infinitely long to us, but in old age, the years just flash by. We compress time with the years due to the relativity of time units to our own age. For a 10-year-old, a year is a tenth of his life – for a 100-year-old, only a hundredth. How would a 1,000-year-old feel about the passage of time? Would he be bored to death when he came to a frenetic standstill? The philosopher Williams refers in this context to an Arthur Schopenhauer belief: 'The shortness of life, so often lamented, may be the best thing about it'.

On the other hand, supporters of Thomas Nagel's 'Death robs us of our possibilities' thesis often object: only dull people are bored. Boredom may be a personality thing. Those who choose the Greenland shark or Highlander scenario ultimately question William's conclusion that too much inner development necessarily leads to the dissolution of one's own identity. On an abstract level in a mind game, this resolution appears coherent. But we may underestimate human curiosity and the ability to learn, should death not deprive us of the possibility of new experiences. In a world of long-living, personality development would not have to be mostly completed at 25, as is the case today. Perhaps a long-life perspective increases the motivation to learn throughout one's life and to change more frequently and fundamentally. Maybe we will continue searching for the new and remain curious in the literal sense of the word because we know that we still have enough time to really live the newly learnt.

If we grew old and remained young, we could learn several professions down to the last subtleties and carry them out with a high level of expertise for decades. We would no longer have to make fundamental decisions about our lives at the ages of 15, 18, or 19, which are currently challenging to revise throughout our life. People with double talents in music and mathematics would no longer have to decide between the conservatory and the Technical University at the age of 20. They could first become a mathematician and later a musician. Studying for senior citizens at the age of 70 would no longer be a stimulating hobby but could be the start of a second career. Maybe we would work much more efficiently or creatively in our third or fourth profession because we could draw on a wealth of experience from other domains.

Some marriages become lacklustre after 30 or 40 years, but the partners do not separate because it doesn't seem to make sense from a life perspective of the remaining 10 or 20 years. Assuming longevity, many may find happiness in serial monogamy, with deep, decades-long partnerships and, in between, phases of sexual freedom. In a world of the long-living, there would most likely be radically different family constellations. Without physical ageing, menopause could shift or disappear altogether. We could still go to the zoo with our great-great-great-grandchildren and look at reawakened woolly mammoths thanks to biotechnology. Or we could simply let off steam in the park like 35-year-old parents with their children today.

We could have siblings who are 50 years younger or 100 years older and develop deeper relationships with them that we do not even know today. In a long life, we may be socially much more inventive because we reinvent ourselves repeatedly without having to cut our psychic roots and build entirely new identities, as Bernard Williams believes. If we had the prospect of having many new, joyful experiences at the age of 70 or 120, the human psyche may very well be able to deal with crises much more resiliently and wouldn't scar early. At the same time, we could fall back on an ever-richer wealth of experience. We may generally be much more motivated to change. We may even fundamentally change our character and become better versions of ourselves. Would such a future not be desirable?

Desires and Futures

For Thomas Nagel, the desire for eternal life is rational. The more experiences we can have, the better. For Bernard Williams, the wish represents a naive assumption. Because we are finite beings, we value the life we are granted. Building on Immanuel Kant's ideas about categorical and hypothetical imperatives, Williams distinguishes between contingent (conditional) and categorical (unconditional) wishes and desires. A hypothetical imperative takes the form 'If you want X, then do Y' – it's conditional on having a particular desire or goal. A categorical imperative, in contrast, commands unconditionally – it tells us what we ought to do regardless of our desires or goals. Williams took this basic logical structure – the difference between conditional and unconditional – and applied it in a new way to human desires and life's meaning.

A conditional desire is situational. We are hungry, so we want to eat something. We don't have enough money, so we want a higher salary. We want Manchester City to win the Champions League because we like the coach or dislike Real Madrid. Comforts and the satisfaction of short-term pleasures usually fall into the category of non-categorical desires: a week in Florida or on the Canary Islands, hot sex with a colleague, a large piece of particularly delicious chocolate cake. Conditional desires change throughout a lifetime. And when life ends, they give little justification for why it might be essential for us as individuals to continue living. They are ultimately independent of the desired length of one's own life.

Categorical desires are profound. We hold them independent of our current circumstances. Frequently, it's the categorical desires about which we as individuals say: life is not meaningful if we don't get the chance to fulfil wishes for ourselves (or others). As human beings, we define for ourselves what categorical wishes are for us. For a composer, it may be the piece of music of his life that inspires the masses. For a dissident, it may be the overthrow of a dictator and people's freedom. For parents, the opportunity to experience how their children find a good, happy life, and for grandparents, how their grandchildren graduate from high school. Categorical wishes and desires often apply to our whole life and thus hold our lives and identities together. In extreme cases, people are willing to die for these wishes if it is the only way to make them come true. It is the unconditional desires that awaken in us the wish to live longer, perhaps infinitely.

For Williams, categorical desires turn into contingent wishes through eternal life. Because we can experience (almost) everything in a long life, Williams says, the desire for the things that are crucially important to us wears off. The result would be endless boredom, with desperate attempts to escape into a hedonism that is no longer one because all stimuli have already been exhausted. In other words: immortality is not desirable, since we might eventually exhaust our categorical desires; leaving only contingent ones wouldn't be enough to make eternal life worthwhile.

The Swiss philosopher and physicist Eduard Kaeser imagines it as 'a never-ending cocktail party among Struldbrugs, with the only remaining urge to have another drink. You can't really enjoy it either, and the other Struldbrugs already annoy you anyway'. Kaeser also believes that categorical wishes give meaning and energy to our lives precisely because they often do not, or only partially come true. Although this sounds plausible, it is also based on the premise that we, as humans, are not sufficiently open to and capable of change.

And this is exactly where the most interesting questions arise in this context. What makes life meaningful versus merely filled with activity? How do different desires relate to our sense of identity and purpose? What happens to us humans if our descendants, or we actually experience such a radical change in life perspectives as longevity researchers and enthusiasts hope? How vast is the plasticity of the human being? Can we really reinvent ourselves again and again? Does our soul remain young, open, and capable of development because our biological system creates the conditions for this? Or will spirit and mind scar and degenerate because biotechnology is only good for the body but bad for the psyche?

CHAPTER 4

WHAT WOULD LONGEVITY MEAN FOR JUSTICE, SOCIETIES, AND THE EARTH'S OVERPOPULATION?

Let's repeat the thought experiment with the three life-extending pills. But this time, it should not be about our individual wishes but social issues. What would it mean for social communities if many or most people lived healthily for 100, 200, 400 years, or even many millennia to infinity?

When I ask this question in mixed-age groups, there is almost always a counter-question: Is social security still secure? Then the group usually laughs. In many minds, the pension formula obviously remains a fixed point of consideration, even if the exercise intends to animate utopian thinking. On the one hand, this is funny, but on the other hand, it is entirely justified and conspicuous. Even without biotechnological breakthroughs, the pension systems are already threatening to collapse with the current increase in life expectancy. But at the same time, it is difficult or impossible for governments to raise the retirement age appropriately without being voted out of office at the next opportunity.

Countries such as Denmark, Finland, the Netherlands, Portugal, and Italy have found a politically clever solution. They automatically adjust the statutory retirement age to the increasing life expectancy. If we can find a corresponding basic social consensus, we will resolve the ongoing political dispute over the retirement age. We need to come to this consensus through a rational decision-making process. Because it is self-evident from an economic point of view that longer lives must also entail longer working lives – at least as long as people do the work and cannot fully delegate it to robots and algorithms. Hence, reorganizing retirement for the working is only for starters.

The prospect of radical life extension raises profound questions about capital accumulation and economic inequality. As individuals live well beyond current life expectancy, compound interest – that powerful force that Albert Einstein allegedly called the eighth wonder of the world – would work its magic over much longer periods. The wealthy would have centuries rather than decades to accumulate returns on their investments, potentially leading to unprecedented concentrations of wealth. Without robust wealth taxes or other redistributive mechanisms, society could face the emergence of a virtually immortal plutocracy, commanding resources on a scale that would make today's billionaires look modest by comparison.

This transformation would likely force a fundamental rethinking of monetary policy and interest rates. The current economic paradigm assumes relatively short human time horizons, with interest rates partly reflecting the trade-off between present and future consumption over a typical lifespan. In a world where people routinely live to 150 or beyond, the natural rate of interest might need to fall substantially. After all, if individuals can reasonably expect to live for centuries, they might be willing to accept much lower returns on their investments, fundamentally altering the time value of money. Central banks would need to navigate this new reality, potentially pushing rates into negative territory as standard policy.

The implications for economic growth are equally far-reaching. Lower interest rates might stimulate investment in long-term projects that would be unthinkable under current time horizons. Imagine infrastructure designed to last centuries or research programmes spanning decades. Yet this could be offset by increased risk aversion among the long-lived wealthy, who might prefer to preserve their capital rather than risk it on innovative ventures. The result could be a peculiar form of economic stagnation: abundant capital but little productive investment, as the effectively immortal rich focus on wealth preservation rather than creation. The challenge for societies would be to harness the potential benefits of extended time horizons while preventing the ossification of wealth and opportunity. The alternative – a society divided between immortal rentiers and mortal workers – would make today's inequality debates seem quaint by comparison, as predicted in dystopian science fiction series. But maybe this outlook is far too gloomy. A very different, optimistic scenario is also plausible. Longevity advocates call it 'the longevity dividend'.

The Longevity Dividend

As healthier individuals remain professionally active into their ninth and tenth decades, what was once seen as a demographic time bomb could become an unprecedented economic opportunity. Extended careers would allow professionals to accumulate deeper expertise, build more extensive professional networks, and potentially generate significantly more wealth over their extended lifespans. This might fundamentally reshape labour markets and educational systems, not for the worse, as often assumed, but for the better.

As discussed in the last chapter, individuals might not follow the traditional pattern of front-loaded education followed by a single career but pursue multiple professional paths over a century-long working life. This could not only be personally enriching but also beneficial to national GDPs. The World Economic Forum projects that this 'multi-stage life' could boost productivity by 10–15 per cent through accumulated expertise alone. Universities might evolve to serve students of all ages, creating new markets for adult education and professional development. Meanwhile, the financial services industry would need to innovate, developing products suited to 100-year investment horizons and multiple career transitions.

The implications for consumption and investment patterns could be equally profound. An economy of healthy centenarians would likely generate entirely new markets and industries. The 'silver economy' could expand far beyond current projections, as active older citizens pursue ambitious projects and investments with multi-decade horizons. Venture capital might see a renaissance, as experienced professionals with substantial capital pursue entrepreneurial ventures in their later years. Real estate markets could transform as people plan for much longer occupancy periods, potentially prioritizing quality and sustainability over short-term considerations. For forward-thinking nations and businesses, this longevity-driven transformation offers a unique opportunity to pioneer new economic models built around extended human potential, rather than traditional retirement patterns. And counterintuitively, a longevity dividend might even pay-off in lower health costs.

In principle, the economic burdens caused by a rapidly ageing population could be lower than they seem at first glance, even if longevity medicine progresses at a mediocre speed. The geneticist Nir Barzilai calls it more modestly an 'old-age return through increasing life expectancy'. Barzilai refers to studies by the British economist Andrew Scott, who calculated that a one-year increase in life expectancy would bring an economic benefit of 38 trillion US dollars for every citizen in the United States with the same average health. An average life extension of 10 years would mean 360 trillion US dollars. Even older people who no longer work but remain active travel, shop, and pay taxes on capital income, among other things.

This calculation can only be applied to a limited extent to a pension system financed according to the principles of redistribution and subsidized by taxes. But with prolonged work biographies and a higher capital share to fund retirement, it is easy to create models in which long lives represent an economic opportunity rather than a grim threat. The situation is similar regarding the financing of the healthcare system.

In scientifically acclaimed long-term studies of 100-year-olds, Barzilai has documented that 'centenarians' incur lower healthcare costs in their long lives than those living to be between 60 and 70 years. This is because the very old often remain mainly healthy for a lifetime and die very old after a relatively short phase of illness, often without the necessary medical support. Short periods of morbidity mean significantly lower costs for healthcare systems. As far as we know today, it is primarily genetic factors, or more precisely: the epigenetically controlled ageing processes in the cells, which promote a long, healthy life with short morbidity. Unfortunately, an exemplary lifestyle is less helpful than we think. Suppose geriatric medicine succeeds in extending the so-called healthspan, meaning life in good health, faster than the lifespan, meaning the absolute age. In that case, we can also finance longevity scenarios with the average age of giant tortoises.

For us, this could mean: in the future, we will live longer and die more quickly.

But who is 'we'? Certainly not all of us.

Biological Class Division

Our thought experiment with the three scenarios is an experiment with many unknowns. That is the point of the exercise. From today's perspective, however, at least one premise is entirely unrealistic, namely that white, yellow, or green pills, such as a few drops of polio vaccine on a sugar cube, are distributed free of charge to all people worldwide by a friendly doctor.

If longevity medicine actually achieves major breakthroughs in the coming years or decades, then anti-ageing agents and fountain of youth gene therapies will be very costly. Most likely, they will be even more pricey than expensive high-performance medicine today. However, many people will probably want to live longer, healthier lives as soon as this is possible. So, will only the super-rich be able to afford the longevity super remedies, or will they only be offered to those who invest in longevity medicine today? It is unlikely that health insurance companies and public healthcare systems could shoulder the costs for the general public. Today, individualized gene therapy applications to cure hereditary diseases cost several million dollars, often for a single syringe.

Of course, there is always hope that innovations will become so cheap after a while that many can afford them. In the 1950s, a black-and-white television was a luxury for the rich. However, the prices of and access to longevity medicine will likely exacerbate the problem of national and international multi-class medicine many times over. At least, this would be the case during a more prolonged transition phase. What would that mean from an ethical point of view?

We cannot compare medical progress to the introduction of TV sets. Assuming longevity drugs will only be available to a new class of the long-living, but not to the mass of mere mortals, would a new 'biological class division' emerge, as Israeli historian Yuval Harari calls it? Life extension only for the rich and powerful could lead to a world where economic inequality is reinforced by biological differences, a division between a biologically enhanced elite and the less affluent who remain biologically unenhanced. This could lead to a new form of social stratification, where the gap between the rich and the poor is not just financial but also biological. A 'godlike' elite, Harari warns, and a 'useless class', could exacerbate inequality beyond anything seen in history. In turn, would this lead to a renewed class struggle in societies, possibly heftier than even Karl Marx could imagine? And would the people of the global South push to the North with such power that today's migratory pressure might seem like a mild premonition in retrospect?

The Canadian biomedical ethicist Walter Glannon argues for a categorical and complete ban on longevity medicine solely because of equal access and opportunities. At first glance, this objection seems worth considering: in a world where longevity is possible for some but unattainable for most, inequality will worsen dramatically.

However, from a moral-philosophical point of view, Glannon's proposed ban is problematic: equality is not fair when it denies some people opportunities simply because they are not available to everyone. Nobody would think of denying cancer patients the necessary surgeries or chemotherapy because patients in Bangladesh in the same predicament have no chance of receiving these therapies. Although there are not enough donor kidneys for all those needing one, the few kidneys available are still transplanted and save lives.

At least in theory, the allocation of scarce donor organs in most societies is not based on market mechanisms, that is, according to the respective financial power, but on a socially negotiated prioritization. This includes, among other things, urgency. If longevity medicine becomes a scarce commodity, the question of medical triage could also arise here: Who needs the white, yellow, or green pill most urgently? Or where would it be most sensibly used from a social perspective? Would scarce longevity pills first be given to exceptionally gifted people who advance society particularly strongly? Or, to get to the heart of it: Which life is worth prolonging, and which is not?

Longevity medicine will pose big questions of the principle of equality and universal human dignity with new drama. Technological progress usually means that a privileged few can reap the benefits of innovation earlier than others. As a rule, you can buy privilege – and this fact can, of course, be perceived as unjust in the sense of distributive justice. But the wealthy early adopters also provide start-up financing before mass consumption. In the second or third step, thanks to the spread of knowledge about technical feasibility, economies of scale in production, and consequently falling prices, more and more people are gaining access.

At least for a longevity medicine that did not entirely defeat death, there is no categorical difference from today's drugs or treatments that prolong individual lives. Physicians who withhold available longevity therapies from patients who desire longevity are probably violating their Hippocratic oath.

This brings us to the most significant ethical challenges that radical advances in longevity medicine would bring: What would be the social or planetary impact if longevity were possible for many or even everyone?

The Ultimate Methuselah Conspiracy

Already today, in many Western societies, more people retire every year as young people come of age. In some countries, more people need care than there are voters under 30. In the United States, the demographic picture is still slightly better, but with little immigration, the ratio of young to old will soon turn here as well. Then here, too, a gerontocracy could be a threat. The domination of the old, where fewer and fewer young people have less and less influence on the political decision-making process, and more and more older people have more and more vote(s) through their mere mass.

What is particularly disturbing about this gloomy picture of the future based on current demographic figures is that not even mediocre advances in longevity medicine are considered. How bad would it be if the many baby boomers who retire today do not die in 30 years but still have many decades ahead of them and then vote for those who can preserve their vested interests? Then the 'Methuselah Conspiracy' would be perfect, which the publisher of the Frankfurter Allgemeine Zeitung, Frank Schirrmacher, presented 20 years ago as a gloomy prophecy.

Schirrmacher is not alone with his 'German Angst'. Even among Anglo-Saxon sceptics of longevity utopias, we can find the argument: social progress needs biological demise – plain and simple. The new is brought into the world by and large by new generations. Throughout their lives, people find it increasingly difficult to recognize when it is time for something new. Like zombie cells that do not want to die, they block the process of social renewal at all levels.

The prospect of significantly extended lifespans could fundamentally reshape human risk calculations, potentially fostering an era of excessive caution. When individuals expect to live for centuries rather than decades, the natural inclination might be to protect one's extended future at all costs. This could manifest in reduced entrepreneurship, more conservative investment strategies, and a general reluctance to engage in activities that carry even modest physical risks. Young people might adopt the more conservative attitudes typically associated with their elders, knowing they have centuries rather than decades to protect.

Yet this tendency towards risk aversion might be counterbalanced by opposite factors that emerge in a long-lived society. The possibility of recovery from financial setbacks over extended timeframes could encourage more patient, long-term investment strategies. As mentioned earlier, scientific research might benefit from researchers who can pursue complex problems over many decades, while the accumulation of human capital over longer lifespans could drive innovation in unexpected ways.

Moreover, the economic imperatives of funding extended lifespans might necessitate continued technological progress and economic growth, forcing societies to innovate despite their inclination towards caution. In that sense, societies with many long-lifers might deal with a supercharged version of the problem ageing societies already experience today. Many conservative, risk-averse individuals have to invest in new ideas and accept radical reforms to sustain long-term prosperity and wealth.

One thing seems for sure: societies under conditions of longevity would have to leave behind the storm-and-stress narrative that only youth is good and valuable to function. Schirrmacher offered an optimistic way out of the dystopia of the Methuselah's conspiracy: if we renew the image of ageing and reinvent our self-image of growing old and the self-limitation associated with old age due to frailty, we can solve social blocks in the future. The accusation of young climate activists against today's ruling generations of boomers is often characterized by the accusation: You are destroying our future. You yourselves will hardly feel the consequences. In a world of the long-living, at least this accusation would no longer be appropriate because then all generations would actually be in the same boat.

In a successful longevity scenario, decision-makers in politics, business, and society would have to be prepared to take much more consistent ecological transformation steps. Because they would be aware that in 100 or even more years, they would still have to lead a good life on this planet. Abstractly speaking: perhaps a society with many long-living people would be better able to think and act responsibly in the long term. This would affect not only ecological but also social issues. At least in capitalist societies, longevity will also significantly increase material inequality. Personal wealth would accumulate not only over decades but over centuries, as we know it today at best from dynasties or the Catholic Church. Another interesting question is: Would more super-rich people voluntarily share their wealth with others?

In a longevity world, there may be significantly more philanthropists like Bill Gates or Warren Buffet, who ignore an expansion of personal wealth as a motivation for one's own actions beyond the age of 60 and make positive social change their purpose in life. Of course, it is also conceivable that the knowledge of death helps with the willingness to share during one's lifetime and, in this way, to develop a positive self-image and to leave for others even after death. If, on the other hand, philanthropy was to decline rather than increase, legislators could reform inheritance tax law and introduce a kind of virtual tax death. In the cycle of today's generations, for example, every 30 years, part of the accumulated wealth would have to be returned to society.

These considerations presuppose that in a longevity world, there will continue to be controlled – or rather controllable – economic growth and that the world economy will not collapse ecologically or socially under the pressure of overpopulation. This may be the greatest danger of a more radical extension of many people's lives.

The Malthusian Total Catastrophe

A few years ago, the ethicist John K. Davis of California State University, Fullerton, with the help of a demographer, carried out model calculations of population development under the conditions of longevity.

In his first scenario, he assumes a life expectancy of 150 years. Each woman has two children – the first at the age of 25 and the second at the age of 75. Under these conditions, the world's population theoretically grows by slightly more than three times within 100 years. Based on today's population, that would be around 25 billion people. With a constant birth rate of two children, the world's population would then stabilize at this level. If humans could live on average to 1,000 years, and every woman had one child at the age of 25 and one at the age of 500, the population would first double rapidly within 75 years. It would then stagnate for 400 years and, after 600 years, settle at its peak at four times the initial population – from today's perspective, at well over 30 billion people.

We cannot know how many people agriculture can sustainably and efficiently feed in a hundred or several hundred years. We do not know whether humanity will have managed to generate energy in surplus for tens of billions of people without producing too much CO_2. Perhaps by then, there will be economic and material cycles that will enable many people to live a healthy, safe, and comfortable life within the framework of the so-called planetary boundaries and end today's resource overexploitation. Perhaps politics, science, and technology will have succeeded in stabilizing the Earth's ecosystem again by then. That is entirely conceivable. But is it likely?

In general, it will also become more difficult for future generations to stay within the planetary limits the more people inhabit the Earth. Based on today's birth rates, the United Nations predicts only moderate population growth to 10.4 billion people by the end of this century. If the global trend of declining birth rates solidifies, the world's population will likely decline again in the twenty-second century. This means that the faster longevity medicine advances, the greater the time pressure for a global social-ecological transformation.

The problem of overpopulation – described by Thomas Malthus in 1798 in his famous essay 'The Principle of Population' and hereafter referred to as the 'Malthusian Catastrophe' – could be the biggest hurdle to whether scenarios with longevity appear desirable. And a rapidly growing world population due to life extension could also lead to the most significant moral dilemmas.

China has long practised a one-child policy against severe and rapid overpopulation. Is it compatible with our idea of humanity to forbid people from having more than one child? John Davis believes the one-child policy makes sense in balancing a Malthusian total catastrophe through longevity medicine and the individual's right to prolong life. However, he makes a necessary restriction: only those who decide to prolong life artificially must do without second and further children. Thus, the individual decision for longevity therapy would be inseparably linked to the question: Is a desire for a larger family categorically important? Or does a very long life with a maximum of one child seem the better option? Hence, many longevity advocates will claim: these two questions are completely irrelevant, especially when asked with such a sceptical undertone as I do here. They claim: longevity is our best bet to save modern humanity from its strange unwillingness to reproduce. Elon Musk, father of seven, is not only one of the loudest voices in this quire. He, and futurists like Ray Kurzweil, are convinced: longevity is a prerequisite for humanity to explore its full potential. Admittedly, John K. Davis' scenarios could prove totally wrong indeed.

Longevity Meets Longtermism

The relationship between longevity and population size is more complex than it might appear at first glance. Population growth (or decline) obviously depends on both birth rates and death rates. Extended lifespans only affect one side of this equation – the death rate. The birth rate remains a crucial variable that could move independently. Several leading longevity researchers and ethicists have proposed scenarios that might help to ease Malthusian fears.

James Hughes, a bioethicist and former executive director of the Institute for Ethics and Emerging Technologies, argues that longer lifespans might actually lead to lower birth rates because people might feel less pressure to have children early or at all if they know they have centuries rather than decades to make this decision. We already see this pattern in the bigger part of the rich world, where increased life expectancy correlates with lower birth rates, dropping in many countries below replacement fertility.

Laura Carstensen, founding director of the Stanford Center on Longevity, suggests that extended lifespans could lead to what she calls 'time redistribution' rather than pure population growth. In this scenario, people might spread their reproductive years over a much longer period, having the same number of children but spaced further apart. This would change the age structure of society without necessarily increasing the total population.

Longevity by definition needs long-term-thinking. This is where biomedical life extension meets 'longtermism' – a philosophical perspective that prioritizes the long-term future of humanity, arguing that the well-being of future generations should be a central concern in decision-making today. The home turf of this school of thought is unsurprisingly Northern California. Peter Thiel, Jeff Bezos, and Elon Musk are its most prominent sponsors, as was Sam Bankman-Fried before he went to prison for a long time. Academic trailblazers of longtermism are a group of Oxford-trained and associated philosophers, namely Nick Bostrom, Toby Ord, and William MacAskill. They see the relationship between longevity and population as part of a broader story about human potential and existential risk.

The core longtermist argument goes like this: humanity's greatest challenge isn't overpopulation but rather ensuring our species survives and thrives long enough to realize its full potential. In this context, they see longevity as serving several crucial functions:

First, longtermists argue that longer lives would allow humanity to accumulate and preserve knowledge more effectively. When scientists, philosophers, and innovators can work for centuries rather than decades, our civilization's intellectual progress could accelerate dramatically. This is particularly important for solving complex, long-term challenges like climate change or space colonization.

Second, they suggest that longer lifespans would naturally encourage longer-term thinking. People who expect to live for centuries might take more serious interest in long-term problems and solutions. This could lead to more sustainable population dynamics, as people would have a personal stake in ensuring resources last for hundreds of years.

The longtermist's view on population itself is quite nuanced. Rather than focusing on absolute numbers, they emphasize population quality – meaning the capacity of humans to solve problems and advance civilization. From this perspective, a smaller population of very long-lived, highly skilled individuals might contribute more to human flourishing than a larger population with shorter lifespans.

This connects to their broader vision of humanity becoming a space-faring civilization. Spearheaded by Musk, longtermists argue that becoming multi-planetary requires both extended lifespans (for long space journeys) and sufficient population to establish viable colonies. They see current declining birth rates in developed nations as a potential threat to this vision and suggest that longevity technology might help maintain optimal population levels for space expansion. In essence, Bostrom, Musk, et al. reframe the traditional Malthusian concerns. Instead of wondering 'Can Earth support ten, twenty or even more billion people?', longtermists ask, 'What population structure would best enable humanity to expand beyond Earth and realize its potential?'

Fair enough. But what would this mean, in the end, for the most essential question of all in the context of biomedical progress: Do you want to live forever?

CHAPTER 5

THE END OF AGEING?

Two decades ago, Nick Bostrom, the great admonisher of existential risks to humanity, published a remarkable essay in the *Journal of Medical Ethics* entitled 'The Fable of the Dragon-Tyrant'. A giant dragon is terrorizing humanity and killing around 100,000 people every day. Most people have come to terms with the terrifying beast. They see its existence as 'natural' and 'necessary'. Some philosophers even argue that the dragon is good for people. Most people also seem convinced that the dragon is invincible. And the few who want to fight the dragon are seen as naive or dangerous, laughed at or marginalized. The allegory is, of course, easy to decipher.

Around 150,000 people die every day, and around 100,000 of these die from age-related diseases. We fight tooth and nail to save a young life but accept 'natural' death as our human destiny, inevitable. And anyone who questions this dogma is considered a heretic, working against nature or even a God-given order. Bostrom sees this behaviour as paradoxical. His fable is, of course, an appeal: let's end ageing. And the fight against the dragon-tyrant is more than a theoretical possibility. From a moral-philosophical perspective, as framed in the fable, this is a human duty.

Rather unusually for contemporary philosophers, Bostrom has an amazing talent for picking up on the right themes at the right time. The dragon-tyrant entered the fictional stage shortly after the first Methuselah Mouse Prize was awarded to geneticist Andrej Bartke at the 32nd Annual Meeting of the American Aging Society. Bartke had altered the genetic material of a rodent named GHR-KO 11C so that certain growth hormones were inhibited. He also administered special insulin and glucose therapy. As a result, the mouse lived for almost five years, or between 180 and 200 years in human terms. The longevity mouse secured heaps of media attention worldwide, and longevity research had experienced a mid-sized Sputnik moment. With the dragon metaphor, Bostrom provided the philosophical justification for why life extension finally had to be pursued with more power and resources.

Death to the Dragon-Tyrant!

'The Fable of The Dragon-Tyrant' became one of the most quoted texts in the philosophical debate on longevity. It resonated strongly with the 'longtermism' school of thought and the closely associated 'Effective Altruism' movement. That is not all too surprising: the core message of Bostrom's is, at least at first glance, all too plausible.

We humans fight with all our energy for every younger or middle-aged life that is on the line, against every small and medium-sized dragon that shortens our lives. But we let the great tyrant play his deadly game unhindered. Since the publication of Bostrom's essay, the attitude towards radical medical life extension has changed considerably. Those who call for it are no longer marginalized as cranks. The people who invest billions in longevity research are usually highly successful entrepreneurs and often highly rational analysts. Even in philosophy and the humanities, Bostrom's stance is no longer a radical minority position.

Yuval Harari's 'Homo Deus' is, self-evidently, a long-lifer and socially acceptable as a vision of a possible transhuman future. At parties in Northern California, as I have experienced on several occasions, you are more likely to be considered a nutcase if you question the desire for longevity, or if you even claim that the dragon-tyrant will continue to wreak havoc and should be doing so for a variety of reasons discussed in the last two chapters. In short: Bostrom's fable has achieved its goal.

The hunt for the dragon-tyrant is on. And many people cheer the dragon slayers. Hence, some might hold too high expectations about the pace of the progress not in the upper spheres of moral philosophy, but the minuscule world of microbiology.

In the course of my research for this book, I spoke to many scientists from the medical mainstream. Most of them believe that the overly grandiose promises of longevity innovators are unrealistic. Most of them do not, for example, believe in the concept of 'longevity escape velocity' and most certainly not in the idea that the first person to live to be a thousand years old has already been born. There is just no scientific evidence for this. In turn, many of the mainstream scientists I talked to consider it a plausible scenario that there will be people who live to be 150 or 180 years old in the next century but shy away from any guesses on how likely this possible future is. Meanwhile, the majority of the clever minds in gerontology I interviewed assume that it will be easier to overcome the physical infirmities of old age than the psychological challenges of living to the age of a giant tortoise. And the sociologically interested among them vacillate at least between optimism and pessimism when it comes to the political and social consequences that a longevity revolution would inevitably entail.

Again: Which Pill Would You Choose?

Let's revisit the thought experiment from the introduction to this book. Do you want to live forever? As a reminder, you have the choice between a white pill that will give you 90 to 100 healthy years. The yellow pill gives you a healthy lifespan like a giant tortoise or a Greenland shark, that is, around 200 to 400 years. The green pill opens the door to physical immortality, let's say at least a thousand years, but perhaps much more. For me, this thought experiment raises two central initial questions that everyone would first have to clarify for themselves before they could make a rational choice in this, from today's perspective, fictional decision-making situation.

1. Individually:

Firstly, do you believe that you personally could reinvent yourself often enough to keep experiencing new things? In other words, that you can maintain your curiosity even in old age and thus might overcome the fast-time effect that old people experience today?

2. Collectively:

Bear in mind that you will not be the only long-lived person, but that societies will have to change radically along with many long-lived people. New societal and planetary realities will emerge. Do you believe that by the end of this century or the next, humanity will be able to solve the major justice issues associated with longevity peacefully, with at least a satisfactory outcome? Do you believe that humanity will be able to use social and technological innovations to feed significantly more people on this planet and ensure their prosperity, while at the same time ending the overexploitation that is currently leading us towards an ecological collapse of the earth system?

Nobody knows the future. It can only be predicted from historic and current data if we are dealing with linear developments. The 'End of Ageing' would be the opposite of linear; at least in this respect, we are on safe ground with the forecast. Biotechnology, invented and applied by humans, would redefine the very essence of human life. So again, which pill would you choose? Not out of the impulse that more is usually better and that you can always choose the exit option in scenarios 2 and 3?

Of course, even from today's perspective, there are many good reasons to see longevity scenarios as desirable futures. However, among the participants in my workshops who opt for the yellow or green pill, I often perceive a good deal of naivety, sometimes coupled with an astonishing dose of egocentricity and self-confidence. Behind the self-confidence, especially in men over 40, there seems to be a barely masked attitude: the world would be worse off without me. In this is the basic assumption: the choice of longevity is only logical, an individual and collective gain. Those who opt for the green pill are generally united by an irrepressible optimism. I often find this unconditional confidence in oneself and the future impressive. Unfortunately, I can't quite go along with that.

I would really like to try the yellow pill. Playing football with great-great-great-grandchildren in the garden sounds very tempting to me. However, after careful consideration, I choose the white one. I see myself as a rational optimist. I am convinced that the world is getting better, and we have plenty of data to prove it, especially in medicine. Progress, no matter how we may exactly define it, is always struggling with setbacks. But it is making progress. For me personally, I would be optimistic that I could remain curious in a young body even at 150. A Beethoven concert was a great experience 200 years ago, just like today. Why should it be any different in 200 years' time, and would we not enjoy a new interpretation of Bach as much as we can today?I am 54 years old today. I decided to become a journalist when I was 16 and, building on that, became a science and tech author and keynote speaker. I will probably do that for as long as I can. But I would also have liked to be an elementary school teacher, as my mother was. And when I talk to scientists who found start-ups based on their scientific findings, I often think that could have been my path too. I'm not going to be a teacher or the founder of a science-based start-up in my lifetime. That's not a personal tragedy. I love what I do. But it might still be missing out, and ideally children could benefit from being taught by me as well. Self-aggrandizement as a long-life chancer aside, my rational optimism does not go as far as to believe that real life extension would be a win-win situation for humanity. I fear a Methuselah conspiracy would be inevitable.

My first big concern is: Who gets access to longevity therapies first? The tech oligarchs who fund them? Or the successors of Putin, Xi, or Trump? What happens when long-lived autocrats try to secure their power forever? Will they unleash even bloodier power struggles and take humanity over the brink to self-destruction? That rather looks likely to me.

Biotechnological longevity harbours a dangerous paradox. Individual life chances for the long-lived will increase the existential risks to humanity. Of course, it is conceivable that humanity will have learnt to master these profound risks as a not only technologically potent, but socially wise species by then, as Toby Ord hopes in his brilliant book *The Precipice: Existential Risk and the Future of Humanity*. But how likely is that?

My second major objection to the yellow and green pill is of a demographic nature. From today's perspective, John K. Davis's scenarios on population growth under the conditions of longevity from the last chapter also seem plausible and even probable to me. This would then also mean that there is a high probability that variants of one-child policies would have to be introduced. They were a meaningful and logical conclusion from the scenarios he calculated. From a social perspective, however, it encounters at least two crucial problems:

First, a law limiting the number of children for long-living people could probably only be enforced in a dictatorship but not in a liberal democracy. Suppose a long-living woman becomes pregnant: Does she have to abort the child? Or suppose that the child is born: Does it then have to lead a life on the margins of society, like the millions of 'illegal' people in China, whose parents, mostly from rural areas, had no right to a second child and could also not buy this right?

Second, a one-child policy logically means that, over the centuries, fewer and fewer children and young people will live in a long-living society. This would not be a desirable future for me, even if low numbers for children in an ageing society did not have to be enforced but happened voluntarily, in continuation of the trends we know today from child-poor societies.

My categorical desires in the sense of Bernard Williams include, firstly, that even autocrats and despots are regularly swept away by death and that biology creates the opportunity for a democratic new beginning. And secondly, that many children and young people live in and refresh societies. I don't want to prolong my life anyway if all the people I love around me die before me. So, if I assume that not only I, but many people, or ideally everyone, could choose yellow and green pills, I can only hope that death cannot be defeated. That there will be no yellow and green pills and that the entropic decay processes of biology will prove to be invincible opponents for us humans with ambitions to become 'homo deus'. I am in good intellectual company with this conclusion.

When Schopenhauer Meets Steve Jobs

'The shortness of life, so often lamented, may be the best thing about it.' The quote comes from the nineteenth-century philosopher Arthur Schopenhauer. For him, death is part of the natural order. It is neither a tragedy nor a problem but simply the way nature renews life. Meanwhile, according to Schopenhauer, fearing death is irrational because we did not suffer before we were born; why should we fear non-existence after death?

Admittedly, Arthur Schopenhauer's thinking was characterized by empirical and metaphysical pessimism. That cannot be said about Steve Jobs. In his famous commencement speech at Stanford University in 2005, the founder of Apple turned Schopenhauer's idea of redemption through death into a logic of personal urgency. Our finiteness of life is an opportunity to enrich our lives. And for Jobs, death was, as a fundamental principle of social renewal, a prerequisite for innovation, the most important driving force of progress. Accordingly, Steve Jobs's central message to the students was:

> Death is the destination we all share. No one has ever escaped it. And that is as it should be. Because death is very likely the single best invention of life. It's life's change agent, it clears out the old to make way for the new. Right now the new is you. But someday not too long from now, you will gradually become the old and be cleared away. Sorry to be so dramatic. But it's quite true. Your time is limited. So don't waste it living someone else's life.

Jobs gave the speech shortly after it had looked as though he would very soon die of pancreatic cancer. Through fortunate medical circumstances, he once again escaped death. After the speech, Jobs had around six years left. He tried alternative medicine and, in the very end, avoided the harshest interventions of high-performance medicine, which could at best have brought a short-term extension of life at the price of prolonged suffering.

Would Jobs have taken the white pill safely? Probably. I've met very few people who wouldn't rather swallow it today than tomorrow. If it comes onto the market in my lifetime, which I don't expect, I will take it without hesitation. In this respect, I wish the dragon slayers of Bostrom's dragon-tyrant rapid partial success on the front line of biomedical progress.

I hope that all the scientific endeavours of longevity medicine, and all the billions venture capital funnels towards life extension, will lead us to age much healthier and shorten what philosopher Martin Heidegger calls the 'run-up to death'. That is that phase of morbidity in which our body clings to life, but we cannot rationally understand why we are not allowed to leave. Against this long run-up, longevity medicine in all its impressive scientific ambition can become a blessing as a desired side effect of the human ambition to conquer death. For utopian assumptions on radical life extension, a healthy dose of scepticism might be a helpful medicine.

LITERATURE AND FURTHER READING

Adler, Yael: Kann man das Alter des Körpers Aufhalten. In *FAZ*, 7 February 2022. https://www.faz.net/aktuell/stil/leib-seele /anti-aging-kann-man-das-altern-des-koerpers-aufhalten -17779288.html

Arrison, Sonia: 100 *Plus. How the Coming Age of Longevity Will Change Everything From Careers and Relationships to Family and Faith*. New York: Basic Books, 2011.

Barzilai, Nir: Wir werden mit 80 und 90 Jahren noch arbeiten. In *Interview in FAZ*, 2 October 2022. https://www.faz.net/aktuell /karriere-hochschule/buero-co/altersforschung-wir-werden -mit-80-und-90-jahren-noch-arbeiten-18350846.html

BBC: David Goodall: Australian Scientist, 104, Ends Life 'Happy'. 10 May 2018. https://www.bbc.com/news/world -australia-43957874

de Beauvoir, Simone: *Alle Menschen sind sterblich*. Dt. Erstausgabe, Hamburg: Rowohlt Verlag, 1949.

Bostrom, Nick: The Fable of the Dragon Tyrant. *Journal of Medical Ethics* 31, no. 5 (2005): 273–277. https://doi.org/10.1136/jme .2004.009035

Čapek, Karel: *Věc Makropulos*. Prague: Aventinum, 1922.

Conese, M., Carbone, A., Beccia, E., Angiolillo, A.: The Fountain of Youth: A Tale of Parabiosis, Stem Cells, and Rejuvenation. *Open Med (Wars)* 12 (2017): 376–383. https://doi.org/10.1515/med-2017-0053

Coughlin, Joseph F. *The Longevity Economy: Unlocking the World's Fastest-Growing, Most Misunderstood Market.* New York: PublicAffairs, 2017.

Davis, John K.: *New Methuselahs. The Ethics of Life Extension.* Cambridge: MIT Press, 2018.

————: Want to Live Longer? Consider the Ethics. In *The Conversation*, 31 August 2018. https://theconversation.com/want-to-live-longer-consider-the-ethics-101301

The Economist: Adding Ages. The Fight to Cheat Death Is Hotting Up. 13 August 2016. https://www.economist.com/briefing/2016/08/13/adding-ages

————: A \$3bn bet on Finding the Fountain of Youth. Can an Instant Unicorn Crack Cellular Rejuvenation? 22 January 2022. https://www.economist.com/science-and-technology/a-3bn-bet-on-finding-the-fountain-of-youth/21807244

Gopnik, Adam: Can We Live Longer but Stay Younger? In *The New Yorker*, Mai 2019. https://www.newyorker.com/magazine/2019/05/20/can-we-live-longer-but-stay-younger

de Grey, Aubrey, Rae, Michael: *Ending Aging. The Rejuvenation Breakthroughs that Could Reverse Human Aging in Our Lifetime.* London: St. Martin's Press, 2007.

Fischer, John Martin, Mitchell-Yellin, Benjamin: Immortality and Boredom. *The Journal of Ethics* 18, no. 4 (2014): 353–372. https://www.jstor.org/stable/43895884

Fukuyama, Francis: *Our Posthuman Future: Consequences of the Biotechnology Revolution.* New York: Picador, 2003.

Fortuna, Harry: What Would Life Look Like if We Lived Forever? In *Quartz*, 24 January 2018. https://qz.com/1186171/what-would-life-look-like-if-we-lived-forever

Glannon, Walter: *Genes and Future People: Philosophical Issues in Human Genetics*. London: Routledge, 2018.

————: Extending the Human Life Span. *Journal of Medicine and Philosophy* 27, no 30 (2002): 339–354.

Eduard Kaeser: Lang, länger, ewig leben – ein Albtraum. In *Aargauer Zeitung*, 24 November 2018. https://www.aargauerzeitung.ch/meinung/kommentare-aaz/lang-langer-ewig-leben-ein-albtraum-ld.1329011

Harari, Yuval: *Homo Deus: A Brief History of Tomorrow*. New York: HarperCollins, 2016.

Kirkwood, Tom: *Time of Our Lives: The Science of Human Aging*. New York: Oxford University Press, 1999.

Loeb, Avi: What if We Could Live for a Million Years? In *The Scientific American*, 16 August 2016. https://www.scientificamerican.com/article/what-if-we-could-live-for-a-million-years/

López-Otín, Carlos et al: Hallmarks of Aging: An Expanding Universe. *Cell* 186, no. 2 (2023): 243–278. https://www.cell.com/cell/fulltext/S0092-8674(22)01377-0?_returnURL=https%3A%2F%2Flinkinghub.elsevier.com%2Fretrieve%2Fpii%2FS0092867422013770%3Fshowall%3Dtrue

MacAskill, William: *What We Owe the Future*. New York: Basic Books, 2022.

Müller-Werdan, Ursula. In Conversation with Thomas Ramge. In *Podcast SPRIND*, 6 June 2022. https://www.sprind.org/de/podcast/34-ursula-mueller-werdan/ (in German)

Nagel, Thomas: Death. In *Mortal Questions*, edited by Thomas Nagel, 1–10. Cambridge: Cambridge University Press, 1991.

Ord, Toby: *The Precipice: Existential Risk and the Future of Humanity.* US edition, New York: Hachette Books, 2020.

Olshansky, Jay S. et al.: The Longevity Dividend: Health as an Investment. *Discussion Paper,* 2016. https://ideas.repec.org/p/mea/meawpa/201216.html

Pew Research Center: Living to 120 and Beyond. New Survey Examines Public's Views on Aging, Medical Advances and Radical Life Extension. 6 August 2013. https://www.pewresearch.org/religion/2013/08/06/living-to-120-and-beyond

Pyrkov, T.V., Avchaciov, K., Tarkhov, A.E. et al.: Longitudinal Analysis of Blood Markers Reveals Progressive Loss of Resilience and Predicts Human Lifespan Limit. *Nature Communicatioons* 12, no. 1 (2021): 2765. https://doi.org/10.1038/s41467-021-23014-1

Ramge, Thomas: *Who's Afraid of AI? Fear and Promise in the Age of Thinking Machines.* New York: The Experiment, 2018.

Ramge, Thomas, Laguna de la Vera, Rafael: *On the Brink of Utopia. Reinventing Innovation to Solve the World's Largest Problems.* Cambridge, MA: MIT Press, 2023. Open Access: https://direct.mit.edu/books/book/5677/On-the-Brink-of-UtopiaReinventing-Innovation-to

Sandel, Michael: *The Case Against Perfection: Ethics in the Age of Genetic Engineering.* Cambridge: Belknap Press, 2009.

Schirrmacher, Frank: *Das Methusalem-Komplott. Die Menschheit altert in unvorstellbarem Ausmaß, Wir müssen das Problem unseres eigenen Alterns lösen, um das Problem der Welt zu lösen.* München: Karl Blessing Verlag, 2004.

Scott, Andrew: The Long, Good Life. In *International Monetary Fund,* March 2020. https://www.imf.org/en/Publications

/fandd/issues/2020/03/the-future-of-aging-guide-for
-policymakers-scott

Sinclair, David A.: *Lifespan. Why We Age – and Why We Don't Have to.* New York: Thorsons, 2019.

Singer, A. Michael: Commentary: What is Aging? Can it be Eliminated? *Current Aging Science* 8, no. 3 (2015): 216–219. https://dx.doi.org/10.2174/1874609808031510271315 48

Singer, Peter: Research into Aging: Should it be Guided by the Interests of Present Individuals, Future Individuals, or the Species? In *Life Span Extension: Consequences and Open Questions*, edited by F. Ludwig, 132–145. New York: Springer Publishing Company, 1991.

Steele, Andrew: *Ageless. The New Science of Getting Older Without Getting Old.* London: Bloomsbury, 2020.

Swift, Jonathan: Gulliver's Travels with an Introduction by Robert J. DeMaria. New York: W.W. Norton & Company, 2003.

Wilde, Oscar: *The Picture of Dorian Gray.* Ware: Wordsworth Classics, 1992.

Williams, Bernard: The Makropulos Case: Reflections on the Tedium of Immortality. *The Metaphysics of Death*, edited by John Martin Fischer, 71–92. Redwood City: Stanford University Press, 2022. https://doi.org/10.1515/9781503622036-007

World Economic Forum: We'll Live to 100 – How Can We Afford It?, In *White Paper*, 2017. https://www.weforum.org/whitepapers/we-ll-live-to-100-how-can-we-afford-it

Who wants to live forever
Who dares to love forever
When love must die
But touch my tears with your lips
Touch my world with your fingertips
And we can have forever
And we can love forever
Forever is our today
Who wants to live forever
Who wants to live forever
Forever is our today
Who waits forever anyway?

Queen

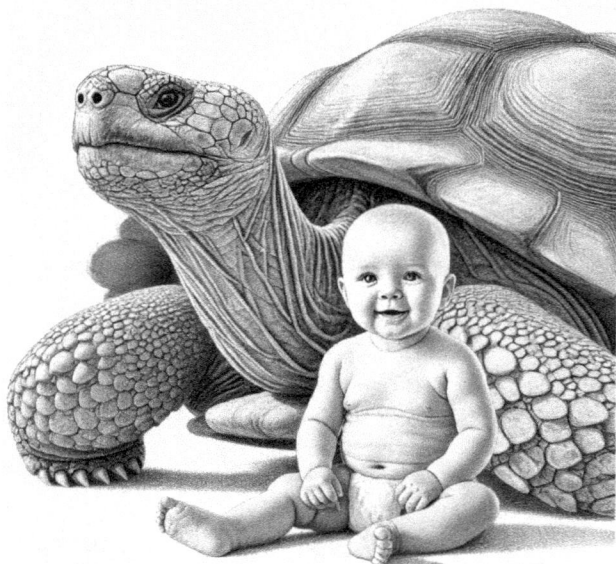